THE RUNNING-SHAPED HOLE

Robert Earl
Stewart

THE RUNNING-SHAPED HOLE

a memoir

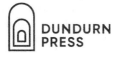

DUNDURN
PRESS

Publisher and Acquiring Editor: Scott Fraser | Editor: Dominic Farrell
Cover designer: Laura Boyle
Cover image: unsplash.com/Birgith Roosipuu

Library and Archives Canada Cataloguing in Publication

Title: The running-shaped hole : a memoir / Robert Earl Stewart.
Names: Stewart, Robert Earl, 1974- author.
Identifiers: Canadiana (print) 20210337230 | Canadiana (ebook) 20210337249 | ISBN 9781459749054 (softcover) | ISBN 9781459749061 (PDF) | ISBN 9781459749078 (EPUB)
Subjects: LCSH: Stewart, Robert Earl, 1974-—Health. | LCSH: Stewart, Robert Earl, 1974- | LCSH: Runners (Sports)—Canada—Biography. | LCSH: Overweight men—Canada—Biography. | LCSH: Weight loss. | CSH: Authors, Canadian (English)—Biography. | LCGFT: Autobiographies.
Classification: LCC GV1061.15.S74 A3 2022 | DDC 796.42092—dc23

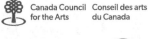

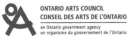
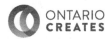

We acknowledge the support of the Canada Council for the Arts and the Ontario Arts Council for our publishing program. We also acknowledge the financial support of the Government of Ontario, through the Ontario Book Publishing Tax Credit and Ontario Creates, and the Government of Canada.

Dundurn Press
1382 Queen Street East
Toronto, Ontario, Canada M4L 1C9
dundurn.com, @dundurnpress 𝕏 f ⊙

For my mother, a promise made.
And for my father, a promise to my mother.

What else does this craving, and this helplessness, proclaim but that there was once in man a true happiness, of which all that now remains is the empty print and trace? This he tries in vain to fill with everything around him, seeking in things that are not there the help he cannot find in those that are, though none can help, since this infinite abyss can be filled only with an infinite and immutable object; in other words by God himself.

— Blaise Pascal, *Pensées*

PROLOGUE

A DEATHBED PROMISE

WHILE SHE WAS lying on her deathbed, my mother asked me to promise her that I would lose weight and get in shape.

But even as she lay there at fifty-eight years old, dying from an insidious *Cytomegalovirus* infection that was devouring her organs, I denied her that promise. I had the gall to make an excuse. Sitting at the foot of her hospital bed that June day in 2006, I looked into her desperate, dying face and told her, "I just don't have the time. I'm just too busy" — too busy being a writer who hadn't really written anything yet; too busy being the editor of a weekly newspaper. I was too puffed up on my own self-importance to realize what a terrible son I was being.

I wasn't a child. I was thirty-two years old. And I sat there in a chair pulled up to the foot of a hospital bed that my mother would never leave, too sad and afraid to make eye contact with the person who had brought me into this world. My father sat at the head of the bed, holding my mother's hand. I heard my name escape his lips, whispered with exasperated disgust.

One could argue that my inability to make that promise to my mother stemmed from my wanting to remain in a state of denial about her health, wanting to pretend, even if only for a bit longer, that my mother was not dying. Making a promise of that magnitude seemed tantamount to admitting that this was, in fact, her deathbed. If I could persist in a state of stubborn self-delusion about my weight, which at the time was topping three hundred pounds, and the impact it had had on my health for years on end, then surely I could also imagine a world where my mother convalesced; where the person I loved did not incrementally disappear from her body; where she did not linger through emergency surgeries in which long tracts of her intestine were removed; where death did not become the best option; where death did not take her from us too soon. Promising something, anything at all, in the dire confines of Intensive Care just seemed too final, too terrifying, too real. Living in that state of denial was a way to insulate myself from my guilt — a guilt I would never be able to escape, of course, as it would descend on me like a shroud of shame whenever I recalled my failure at the foot of her hospital bed, which was often.

"That's no kind of answer," said my father, once my mother had closed her eyes and slipped into over-drugged unconsciousness. His own eyes were puffy and red with grief. We were only a week into what would become a torturous five-month decline. "Would it kill you just to make a little effort?"

I wanted to tell him that it might but knew this was not the time. "I just don't know when I would fit it in," I whined. "Getting in shape? That's a lot of work, and I've got the newspaper, and the boys, and Jen and the baby …" I was quickly out of excuses, and my excuses were all excellent reasons to put some effort into my health — both physical and mental.

Everyone knows the sound their father makes when he is disgusted with you — for failing to clean up your bedroom, for having your second bike stolen in a single summer, for being caught with a dubbed cassette copy of the Beastie Boys' *Licensed to Ill*, for coming home drunk for the fifteenth time in high school ... That was the sound he made then as he turned away from me to place a cool cloth to my mother's fevered brow.

"That's all she wants from you, Bobby," he said, choking back sobs. "She wants you to be happy and healthy. Apparently, that's *too much*, though."

What would have been the real harm, I've always wondered, in saying "Okay, Mom, I promise," whether I meant it or not, when hanging in the balance was some thread of hope and happiness for a terminally ill woman: a vision of her adult son, healthy and hale, instead of the bloated gastropod slumped in embarrassment at her perfect feet. The harm, I knew, was that if I promised to lose weight, to exercise and eat right — promises I had made to myself many times, in vain — I might actually have to make some monumental changes, whether she lived to see them or not.

So, I stayed "too busy."

She was too weak to argue with me, but my mother wore her deep disappointment and her sadness on her face. She may not have been able to eat, but she could still be mad at her son.

o   o   o

Flash forward to November 2012. I'm driving northbound on Howard Avenue in Windsor. I'm thirty-eight years old. I weigh 368 pounds. I've just left an appointment with a cardiologist, and I'm crying my eyes out behind the wheel of my minivan. My mother has been dead for six years. She slipped away on an October day in 2006 while my dad walked from the hospital to their nearby home to eat supper. At the time, I was likely fresh in the door from work at the newspaper, on my hands and knees digging a Luke Skywalker action figure out from under our old upright grand piano with a school ruler. The phone rang; my wife, Jennifer, answered and after a too-brief conversation handed me the phone. The tears of what she feared was true rolled from her eyes while our son Nathanael, four at the time, stood looking up at me while I listened to my crying father tell me my mother was gone.

But I'm not in tears at the thought of my mother, nor am I in tears because I can barely fit behind the steering wheel. I'm in tears because I want to go to my favourite restaurant and eat my face off, and I'm in tears because I am realizing something — something crucial.

My visit to the cardiologist hadn't been a social call. For months, I'd been out of breath, dizzy, and increasingly immobile — those were just the obvious physical symptoms. I was also depressed and scared out of my mind that I was too far gone; that failure to promise my mother that I would lose weight had poisoned my soul; that my selfishness and my gluttony would not only kill me, they would result in me dying a disgrace in my mother's eyes. The only thing that would make me feel better in the depths of all of this self-loathing and self-pity was stuffing myself sick with food, ignoring the fact that the reason I was leaving a cardiologist's was that I was eating my heart right out of commission.

I'm realizing I have reached some kind of crisis point.

My troubles had started several months earlier when I began noticing I was having trouble breathing while talking. Even speaking at regular, conversational volumes, I was running out of air; mid-sentence, I would just peter out. But after recovering with some gasping breaths, I would just dismiss it as some kind of acute, one-off anomaly before continuing. The very act of talking, something journalists have to do *a lot of* as part of their jobs, was becoming too much for me. I would sweat freely just speaking aloud.

4

Once I became conscious of it, I started to worry obsessively about it. One night, I was asked to read aloud at a meeting I attended with some other recovering alcoholics. Following the meeting, two older women approached me and asked if I was okay; they said it had seemed as if I was struggling to breathe through the entire reading. I acted surprised and suggested that maybe my allergies were to blame. They weren't buying it. One of them suggested that maybe I should see a doctor, that my colour wasn't good. Now, other people were not just noticing that I was losing my breath while talking; they were calling me out on it and telling me that something was wrong. They were forcing me to get honest, to stop blaming my seasonal allergies for an inability to breathe. I knew what the problem was, obviously. My lungs were having trouble expanding — unsurprising, given the large amount of weight piled on top of them; my heart was having trouble pumping blood to my muscles and tissues and organs. I was on the verge of some kind of respiratory collapse: an infarction, a heart attack, cardiac arrest.

I was now willing to consult a doctor. Still, I was hoping against hope that a medical professional would confirm that allergies were the cause of my breathing problems. Maybe they would even go further, maybe they would compliment me on carrying my weight well — for years I had been telling people I weighed "about three hundred and ten pounds," but truth be told, I had no idea how much I weighed at this point, since our digital bathroom scale said I weighed "Err," for "Error," because it maxed out at 340 pounds — and send me on my way with a fresh lollipop.

Dr. Hanson didn't tell me any of that. She listened to my heart and lungs impassively. She took my blood pressure and frowned. She weighed me and clucked in disapproval. She had only been my doctor for a short time (following the retirement of the man who had been my doctor since birth, Dr. Sijan), but in less than a year, she had seen me pack on a lot of weight.

When she made the referral to the cardiology centre, she told me that on the day of my appointment I needed to dress in "active wear," which made me think of the tracksuits the old Italian men wear while sitting in front of the cafes along Erie Street. And although the thought of sporting racing-striped velour active wear coordinates pleased me to no end, seeing the mismatched track pants and sweatshirt combos I used for writing and lounging about the house laid out on the bed, freshly laundered, made me wonder who wore such comically outsized clothes.

"Whose pants are those?!" I said one morning, gesturing at a giant square of fabric spread out over the end of our bed.

"Those are yours, honey," Jennifer would say, gently. "Your navy tracksuit ones? I just brought them up from the laundry."

I stared, incredulous. "They look like a flag ready to be draped over a coffin!" I said, approaching them cautiously. "I don't look like someone who needs to wear those pants, do I?"

"Don't say that," Jennifer said, putting a hand on my chest. "You don't have to wear them forever, you know. Make today *the day*. I know we say it a lot, but we can both eat better and get more exercise. I will help you …"

But I wasn't listening. I was looking in the bedroom vanity mirror, appraising myself. "I don't look like that guy we see walking sometimes, do I? I'm not that big, am I? Oh man, don't even tell me. Maybe it's just because they're laying flat and not, like, around my circumference, you know?"

Scenes like this played out in our home with alarming frequency. And every time I would come to the shattering realization that these were indeed my clothes and that they were probably on their way to being too small.

Having occasion to put them on and wear them outside of the house only ratcheted up my self-loathing. The blown-out, New Balance running shoes that I had purchased in the zeal of some short-lived past attempt to lose weight and get healthy really brought the whole ensemble together.

"They are going to do an echocardiogram, an ultrasound of the heart, and put you on a treadmill," Dr. Hanson had told me. I was terrified. I was going to expire in a ghastly heap on that treadmill. In my head, I was always expiring in ghastly heaps — at my desk in the editorial bullpen; in a canoe with my children looking on, horrified; trying to tie my shoes or looking for a book on a low shelf; in the act of lovemaking, traumatizing my wife and anyone with whom she cared to share the whole sad story.

I knew this stress test was going to be a death march, but I was gamely going to show up for the appointment, get on the treadmill, and show the team at Windsor Cardiac Centre how to die a sober disgrace.

"He died trying to get healthy," they would crow down at Kurley's AC, where I used to drink and eat myself insensate some nine years earlier. "He had a big heart," some wag would say at my funeral. "A really big, stressed-out heart."

I'd taken the entire day off work, even though Dr. Hanson had told me my appointment at the cardiologist's would only take an hour. I took the whole day off work so I could rest, focus on bringing my heart rate down, and sort out my personal affairs.

My appointment was for 11:30 a.m. on November 28, 2012. I entered the waiting area, resplendent in the mismatched tracksuit that Jennifer had lovingly assured me I looked "very handsome" in. Checking over my appointment information, the receptionist confirmed that I was here for an echocardiogram but *not* a stress test.

"But I wore these ridiculous track pants and this zip-up windbreaker because my doctor said I would be getting on a treadmill," I protested, not wanting all of my pre–stress test stress to be for naught.

No, the receptionist informed me, the stress test was booked for another day — January 3, 2013, nearly five weeks away. I sat in the waiting room, feeling duped, deprived of my opportunity to face up to my fate by the scheduling vagaries of the health care system.

I'd had ultrasounds before — of my heart, my guts, and, of course, my liver — but this echocardiogram hurt quite a bit more, as the young female technician had to all but climb up on top of the examination table next to me in order to press the transducer into my flesh hard enough for the soundwaves to penetrate both tissue and bone. My sternum and ribcage were creaking like the timbers of an old ship that was being lashed by a storm. They wiped the cold sonogram gel off my chest with a rough paper towel. I was told the results would be discussed with the cardiologist when I came in to do the stress test in January.

I was back out in the parking lot by a few minutes after noon. I hadn't eaten a thing that morning because stress and worry aggravated my various gastrointestinal complaints. I had the rest of the day off and figured I might as well go and get lunch.

Lunch is normally a relatively ordinary affair, unless you're an out-of-control eater lumbering across the Windsor Cardiac Centre parking lot, struggling to catch your breath before you heave yourself behind the wheel of your van. I wasn't planning to settle on a salad and a bottle of mineral water. My appetite was demanding that I sate it with my standard order at Motorburger: a double Firebird burger, a large order of onion rings, and a couple of milkshakes. All of that wolfed down, shamelelssly, right there at the bar, before heading home to sleep the rest of the day away. Inevitably, I would wake up with horrible gastrointestinal complaints and chest pains. This was how you went about a day off work. You got your appointments out of the way early, and then you went out and ate yourself sick. This was normal for me. This was living.

I was driving down Howard Avenue, northbound toward Motorburger on Erie Street, wondering if maybe I should grab a deep-fried dill pickle appetizer with my order, when I realized I was crying. This wasn't lunch. This was a gastronomic suicide mission. I was coming from a cardiologist's office because I could not breathe properly; because I could not carry on normal conversation without running out of air; because I could not get up off the floor unaided if I was down there playing with my children. I was only thirty-eight, and I was scared for my life. Yet, I was driving directly — with avidity — toward the very thing that was killing me, the one thing I was unwilling to let go of in sobriety.

There is very little difference between leaving a cardiology appointment and driving to a restaurant to stuff your face, and leaving a recovery program and driving to a bar to get drunk. It was a compulsion I could not control on my own; a disease arising from my physical reaction to food, my obsessive thinking, and the spiritual hole that resided within me. And as I drove through the city, crying my eyes out, I was just beginning to see it.

I had reached that jumping-off point: where the only thing that would make me happy, the only thing capable of releasing me from the pain and embarrassment of weighing 368 pounds, was eating myself sick. But the reason I was so desperately sad and full of self-loathing was that I weighed 368 pounds from overeating to achieve that all too temporary feeling of, not fullness or satiety, but *peace* — the peace of comfort and familiarity I found in food.

It was no secret to me that this compulsion, this cataclysm of self-consciousness and *self-will*, was itself a symptom of a larger sickness — it was a character defect I was well aware of after nearly a decade of sobriety, and something I was unwilling to change. As a recovering alcoholic, I understand self-will is a diseased manifestation of willpower. I understand that most people believe willpower to be a virtuous, constructive force; the kind of assertive, self-directed stick-to-itiveness touted by self-help gurus, self-styled captains of industry, and well-meaning people the world over. But

I think of it as something very different. In my recovery and in the recovery of many others, the unorthodox definition is the one that holds true.

You don't have to look very far to see that many major religions and philosophical schools of thought warn against the perils of willpower. It is the driving force that keeps an alcoholic actively pursuing their demise, one drink at a time. It is what allows the alcoholic who hates every aspect of their life and being, who knows that alcohol has alienated them from everyone who loves them and has put them, seemingly, well beyond the reaches of hope and help, to continue to get up every day and repeat the humiliating routine, the degenerate behaviour that has brought them to this lowly state. This is not due to some lack of moral fibre, decency, or intelligence in the alcoholic. People will say "He wants to quit; he just lacks the willpower." But what most people do not understand is that it takes near inhuman levels of willpower, dredged up from unfathomable depths, to continue on, to force another drink down, in the face of the overwhelmingly tragic evidence of the pain and suffering their drinking is causing. For those who have suffered alcoholism's ravages and recovered, the word *willpower* is shorthand for the very pathology of the disease of alcoholism — a disease of the mind, body, and spirit that harnesses the will to its progressively fatal ways. It is willpower that kills the alcoholic. It is this perverted sense of willpower that applied to my drinking, and it applied just as aptly to my rapacious appetite.

If it seems like I was having a moment of clarity right there in traffic on Howard Avenue, I *was*. I had become the type of guy who made deathbed excuses to his mother, rather than promises. She didn't want perfection. She just wanted change for the better for her son. And I had denied her.

I'd hit bottom before, and leaving the cardiologist's that day, I knew that I had managed to find another one. Driving down

Howard Avenue in tears because you feel you have no choice; because you feel you're being compelled to drive to a restaurant where you will be an active participant in your own embarrassing, untimely, and unseemly death — *that* qualifies as a low point.

I was so sick of myself. This kind of self-destructive thinking and behaviour was supposed to have disappeared or greatly dissipated after nine-plus years of sobriety, wasn't it? But just as I'd lay in bed in April 2003, ill and isolated and feeling utterly hopeless as a result of my alcoholism — despite having a wife who loved me and was worried sick about me; a wife who went off each morning earning the entire family income single-handedly, while our seven-month-old son was shipped off to a babysitter we couldn't afford because I didn't feel like I could properly take care of him — it wasn't until I got to this terminally low point of fighting the maniacal compulsion to eat that I was able to realize that I had been wrong about almost every aspect of my life up to that moment.

My best thinking had gotten me obese and desperate; no one was going to come along and fix this for me. I had to do something different, something contrary to what my diseased instinct told me was the right thing to do.

Doing "something different" had helped me find sobriety from alcohol. Now, maybe doing the last thing I wanted to do on my day off — something that made me *uncomfortable*; something that made me *fearful* — might just be the best thing for me. I knew from past experience that once you found the bottom, once you have nowhere left to go, you have found the ability, once again, to choose.

I didn't go to Motorburger. I ended up parked on Devonshire Road, near the northeast corner of Willistead Park. It was a wet, grey, blustery day. Instead of going to the restaurant, I made the choice to go for a walk. I headed west on Niagara, turned south down Chilver, circumnavigating the park counter-clockwise not once, but *twice* — a distance, one that is seared in my mind, of 2.2 kilometres.

When I got home, I kicked off my shoes and, ripping off one piece of clothing at a time, stripped myself naked as I hauled myself up the stairs. I faceplanted on the bed, slick in a full body sweat. My head was wreathed by a palimpsest of stains on my foul pillow, subjected as it was to the horrible night sweats I suffered as the result of my weight, my sleep apnea, and sleep apnea's attendant face masks, head gear, and tanks of humidified air. I was out for a few hours.

It's amazing what two trips around the park at a leisurely walking pace will do for you — for starters, if you weigh 368 pounds, it will work you into a lather and take you to the very limits of your physicality — because when I awoke from my nap, something had clearly changed. When Jennifer arrived home from work an hour later, she could *tell* something had changed. She asked how my visit to the cardiologist went, but I was too excited to talk about trifling medical appointments.

"That? That was fine," I said. "But something really big has happened. *At the park.*"

Jennifer was looking at me with an expression of bewilderment and concern that was all too familiar to me — a look from the past: *Was I having a breakdown? Had I been drinking?*

"What happened at the park?" She looked into the living room, where the children sat on the carpet watching after-school television. "What are you talking about?"

"I went for a walk …" I said, amazed at how foreign this admission sounded coming out of my mouth. "I went for a walk around the park. *Twice.*"

I took my wife by the shoulders and looked into her eyes and serious as the heart attack I never wanted to have, said, "I'm done. I'm done with food. I'm done being overweight."

Instead of going to that restaurant I had made the choice to go for a walk. And by making the choice to go for a walk, I had, somehow, made good on my failure to make a deathbed promise to my mother.

Little did I know I'd also made the choice to run.

CHAPTER ONE

THE CONSUMPTION

MY FRIEND SEAN'S parents were out of town, and Sean's crazy uncle Derek was watching his nephews for the weekend. We were a pack of ninth graders, sitting around watching *Charles in Charge* reruns, when Derek announced he was going to the beer store and asked if we wanted anything.

Earlier that day, I'd been fired from my job at the Windsor Farmer's Market. Before dawn on Saturday mornings, my parents had been driving me to the giant, yellow, concrete market building downtown, where I would work at the Scherer's Produce stall until close. I was always a big, strong kid. By grade nine, I was playing high school football, lifting weights, and tipping the two-hundred-pound mark. Because of my size, I was good at the part of the job that required me to stevedore crates of fresh fruits and vegetables around all day. But my mental math skills were questionable at best, and because of my youth and inexperience, I lacked the knack for bartering selling produce requires. I made a lot of mistakes, and I was costing Scherer's either money, or customers.

At the end of a particularly arduous and error-riddled Saturday, I was pulled into the plywood office, given an envelope with my standard forty dollars pay, and told not to come back.

I thought my parents were going to kill me. My father, a long-time Scherer's customer, had gotten me the job. But when I got home and told them what had happened, my parents understood. I think they had probably been tipped off that this was coming. Who knows, maybe my dad was one of the customers I'd either short-changed or given a screaming good deal on green seedless grapes. Either way, my parents slipped me a ten-dollar bill after supper and told me to go out and have a good time with my friends.

So, there we were, being offered alcohol by the coolest adult I knew — Uncle Derek. He was in his midtwenties; he was tattooed; had a show at CJAM, the university radio station; he helped get us in to screenings of *Stop Making Sense, Koyaanisqatsi,* and *The Rocky Horror Picture Show* at the Park Theatre when it was a dilapidated rep house; he let me borrow his Dead Kennedys, the Clash, and Public Image Ltd. albums; and had allegedly been hit with buckshot from a shotgun blast while running down an alley in Detroit.

As a fourteen-year-old who had just been fired from his first job, I was primed to accept the offer of alcohol; it seemed like the perfect adult response to what I viewed as an obvious injustice; it was a salve for my nascent world-weariness. No one else had any money. I pulled the ten-dollar bill my parents had given me out of my pocket and handed it over. Uncle Derek returned a little while later with a full case of premium beer for himself, and a six pack of Old Vienna for us (it was 1989 and a six pack of beer cost about six dollars).

"You can't drink it here, though" he said, withholding the clinking box from our nervous hands. "Connie's coming here after work. You guys gotta split."

So, we went and stood in the freezing February cold behind Walkerville Collegiate, our high school, and drank our two beers each. Standing there in the brick-walled alcove known as the "Smoking Area," I experienced the mood-altering effects of alcohol for the first time. And it was only once that effect had taken hold that I had the courage to confess to my underaged *confrères* what had happened to me earlier that day.

"I got fired from the market today," I said, interjecting my news into a conversation about girls, schoolwork, and music. Silence. "They said I was too young. That I wasn't good at math."

"You fucking suck at math," Sean said.

It got quiet. Snow crunched under out feet. Wind howled across Willistead Park and ice clicked in the trees. It had felt good getting the secret shame of my termination off my chest; there had been a brief respite from self-consciousness, but now I felt that I'd brought the room down.

"Were your parents pissed?" asked Brad, the third member of our drinking party.

"No, they gave me the money I bought the beer with," I said.

We laughed for a long time in the cold and the wind and the dark. There was probably some kind of toast, some kind of pledge of comradery. We were men. Drunk fourteen-year-old men with a purpose.

We went to a nearby house party we'd heard about, and I didn't slow down or look back for fourteen years.

○ ○ ○

Right away, alcohol did everything for me that I could not do for myself. Two beers was all it took. Gone was my native self-consciousness. I felt confident, funny, cool, handsome ... all the things I imagined an adult must experience. Drinking instantly gave me a new personality, providing the key to a social strata that, on my own, I was too introverted to infiltrate.

I wasted no time in putting the distinct fear of raising an alcoholic son into my non-alcoholic parents' hearts. I did not get caught drinking that first night. Nor did I get caught the second time I drank, or the third. But within a month I came home from a party and vomited prodigiously and with a violent roar all over the upstairs bathroom I shared with my younger sister. She just stood in the doorway, crying, looking at me there, sweaty and reeking and bombed on the tile in a room spattered with barf.

"Your sister thought you were dying last night," my mother said the next day, once I was able to get out of bed. "She was terrified. *We* were terrified. We didn't sleep, sitting up making sure you didn't choke to death on your vomit." Now she was crying. "I don't ever want to see you like that again. The people you were with — those older boys who bought you that beer — your father is going to be talking to their parents ..."

Apparently, in my vomitous inebriation, I had given the names of the older students who had been at the house party I had attended the night before — none of whom had anything to do with the six pack of beer I'd consumed, nor the shots of Southern Comfort. When I heard their names repeated back to me, I didn't hesitate — I stuck to my story, happy to throw random high-school seniors under the bus of opprobrium to avoid my parents finding out that I was mature-looking and suddenly confident enough to walk into a beer store and purchase alcohol for myself without ID, real or faked (again, it was the late '80s). Clearly, there would be some fallout for naming names in the delirium of the moment, but nothing that couldn't be smoothed out by purchasing alcohol at some later date for those wrongly fingered innocents who would suffer the consequences following what would almost certainly be my father's apologetic and mannered phone call to their parents.

In the home I grew up in — a home where responsible, occasional social drinking had been modelled by two very gentle and responsible adults — the consequences of my drinking were steep. I was often grounded for months at a time. Inevitably, though, as soon as I was freed from my bondage, I would drink at the first available opportunity. And on more than one occasion I would be caught drunk once again after just mere hours of freedom.

Through all of this, I managed to be an honour-roll student, athlete, and an active member of the student body. By the end of that first year of high school, when it came time for everyone to sign everyone else's yearbook, I was thrilled to see all the messages that identified me as a drinker and a good guy with whom to party.

How my parents felt about me, and what was happening to me as the result of my obsession with alcohol — shifting social priorities; a turning away from the values that I had been raised with; the copping of an outlandishly outsized ego; the unleashing of hedonistic appetites; and, although I wasn't aware of it yet, the courting of a whole slew of new habits that marked the beginning of my gradual slide into full-blown alcoholism — was of little consequence.

My teenaged drinking lent me a good rep in high school, but it was something else that helped to make me "cool" — that mythic quality of dubious meaning: being in a band. From obsessing over my parents' Beatles LPs when I was four years old; to discovering I could tune in the university radio station, CJAM, on an old wooden radio my dad gave me when I was twelve; to taking the bus downtown to buy Black Flag and Deja Voodoo records and taking photos with my dad's Canon Ex Auto at hardcore punk shows held in warehouses and weird ethnic halls around town … music factored heavily into the persona and life I was trying to build for myself.

Little needs to be said about the strong historical relationship between rock and roll and alcohol.

Not surprisingly, as alcohol opened up previously barred social and subcultural doors, introducing me to increasingly non-mainstream and avant-garde music, I was also introduced to the attendant substances that make all that music sound that much more interesting — magic mushrooms and blotter acid with fanciful codenames like "Checkerboard," "Black Magic," and "White Clinical." But while those things came and went, based on capricious circumstances, like who knew a tripped-out stoner just coming off-tour with the Dead, pot was always around in abundance.

From the night I was first introduced to a ball of hashish burning on the end of a pin at a party, to those first glittering nuggets of marijuana in the bottom of a sandwich bag at a different party — alcohol and cannabis in all its forms went together in my life like peanut butter and jam. And if this depressive/hallucinogenic sandwich helped me establish some small space for myself, being in a band — a band that wrote, recorded, and performed its own music — was like a mainline of medical-grade self-confidence and status for an introverted teenager who, left to his own nature, was uncertain about how to get on in the world.

We started out in the summer of 1988, practising in Pat Robitaille's basement. Sean knew Pat from the neighbourhood skateboarding scene; Pat's parents apparently didn't mind the racket. Pat had a broken-down drum kit he couldn't play; I had a Les Paul copy and a little amp and no discernible talent for guitar; and Sean had a Strat, a Fender Princeton Chorus amp, and had been taking lessons. We had no PA system, and we had no songs. I thought I should probably be the singer but was too shy to sing if anyone was around. We called ourselves Chronic Happiness. If there was more to being in a band, we weren't really sure how to achieve those things.

After fumbling around for a few years, during which we talked more about being in a band than we did anything actually musical, Pat switched to bass, we changed our name to Sun Dogs, and John McArthur joined the band.

John's older sisters had been talking him up, telling us for months that their brother was a great drummer. They were right. When John joined the band, there was a dramatic shift in our work ethic — suddenly, we were writing tons of original material and practising several evenings per week — and in our attitude. Tall and lithe, with a chiselled jaw and waves of long blond hair, John was the kind of guy who would show up at school wearing jean shorts, steel-toed work boots with no laces, and a leather jacket with no shirt underneath — and a cigarette tucked behind his ear for good measure.

We were something of a sight to behold for a high-school band: John always on the brink of some kind of fashion meltdown/break-through; Sean, towering six-and-a-half feet, with his shoulder-length blond mane and growing arsenal of guitars; Pat, a wild-eyed skater with a sense of humour as twisted as his maniacal smile; and me, bookish, bespectacled, sporting a mop of dark curls, dread-locks, or a number three crop depending on the season, and a plaid flannel under a black flight jacket.

After about six months of rigorous rehearsing, we'd built up a set list of originals and were booked as the opening act for a Rush-influenced prog rock band at the Coach & Horses — ground zero for the Windsor music scene in the early '90s. None of us was of age, but no one was checking the IDs of the band members. It was free drinks into the wee hours as we became regulars on stage and at the bar, building up a following. Our sound was punishingly loud but melodic and hooky; the stage show intense and chaotic: think Screaming Trees, the Afghan Whigs, Fugazi.

o o o

In all my years in school, I was only able to enjoy one snow day — in January 1992, an epic storm buried Windsor under a blanket of knee-deep powder. With school cancelled, Sean and I agreed to go out looking for hapless motorists who needed a push out of the snow. Ours wasn't an act of pure altruism, however; our hope was that we would earn enough money in tips from grateful motorists to buy a case of beer and two packs of smokes.

It turned out to be a more memorable day than we had planned.

I trudged the kilometre south from my parents' house on Iroquois Street to Sean's dad's big Tudoresque manor in the very heart of Olde Walkerville. On my arrival, I discovered none other than Uncle Derek sitting in the breakfast nook drinking a coffee. He complimented us on our plan to help people in order to earn enough money to get drunk. He also expressed his kudos for a recent Sun Dogs set he'd taken in with a bunch of his CJAM *confrères* at the Coach & Horses.

"You know who you guys should talk to is my buddy Andrew," Derek said. "He's got a studio. He'd really dig you guys." Sean and I were all ears. "Yeah, he's just up at the corner of Wyandotte and Walker. You'll see an iron staircase leading up the side of the building to a door. Just tell him I sent you."

A dark Chevy van was parked in the small lot beneath the iron staircase, nestled in the shadows of the red-brick towers of the Hiram Walker & Sons whisky warehouses. The van hadn't been brushed off since the storm, and the stairs were ascending tiers of undisturbed snow.

We climbed the stairs and thumped on the dented steel door. We stood there waiting in the wind. We thumped again. We smoked a cigarette. We thumped some more. It had just reached the point where if someone actually came to the door it was going to be embarrassing when the door lurched open and a man with long black hair and piercing blue eyes stared out at us.

"Hey," he said uneasily. "What's going on?"

"Derek Jupp sent us. We're in a band. We're looking for a place to record."

He looked us up and down, nodding, then looked over the railing behind us at his van below. "You guys help me brush off the van so I can get to the beer store, and we can come back and talk."

A welder by trade, Andrew was about ten years older than us. He rented the space, and though he wasn't supposed to live there, he did, which is exactly what Sean and I would have done because it was the coolest place either of us had ever seen. From where we stood in the mixed kitchen/welding shop/guitar and amp repair workshop in the front of the space, I could see into long, high-ceilinged room that ran about thirty metres to a glassed-in vocal booth that was lit from above by a skylight. The main room was divided up into a lounge area with sectional couches and coffee tables; a bar, a dining area complete with matching table and chairs; and an area with various drum kits, around which stacks of amplifiers, FX units, mics, stands, guitars and PA systems were situated in what were clearly practice spaces staked out by other bands.

Popping the tops off beers, Andrew passed a couple over to Sean and me. "Wait, are you guys old enough? No? Oh well, it's a snow day!" he said, clinking bottles with us before leading us on a tour.

He pointed out the various pieces of studio gear, a tiled industrial washroom with pristine acoustics, and just off the sunlit vocal booth, a low, dark control room in the middle of which sat an enormous 1970s-vintage Studer mixing console, surrounded by myriad rack units and a huge Tascam reel-to-reel tape machine. It was called Neitherworld Studios. It was the real deal. And it was about to become our base of operations for the next three years.

Within a few days of that initial tour, we moved all our gear into the studio. And after a few rehearsals with Andrew present so he could get a handle on our sound, we were ready to start recording. We were often there late into the night, the control booth filling up with clouds of dope and cigarette smoke, every flat surface a forest of green and brown glass.

Andrew would not accept a penny for his services. He was happy to be putting Neitherworld to use, and he was into what we were doing. He became our studio and live-sound engineer, stage tech, driver, and, despite the age difference, our friend.

The result of that first recording session was a self-titled cassette of twelve original songs that we began selling at our shows, some of which were now taking place in Detroit, and several hours up the highway in London, Kitchener-Waterloo, and Toronto. Looking back, I'm not sure how my parents got any sleep during those years, knowing their seventeen-year-old son and his friends were bombing up and down the 401 in a van driven by a high-pressure welder, having polished off as many complimentary pitchers of beer as the bar he'd played in would allow. But I was still active at school, I was still playing football, I was constantly reading novels, and it seemed that I was a shoo-in for university ... Being a gifted student was a very convenient smokescreen. My marks were high, and so was I.

In the summer of '92, Andrew upgraded some of the recording equipment in the studio: a new reel-to-reel machine and a state-of-the-art DAT machine for mixing down from analogue to digital.

"You know what we should do," he said one night while Sun Dogs were wrapping up practice, "we should re-record your whole album. It will be way better."

We probably cheered like children at a birthday party. The results were so much heavier — the production quality was that much sharper, the songs were that much punchier, the mastering was that much more precise. Our proficiency as musicians was so much better too — they were the same songs, but it was as if we were a new band.

We decided to change our name. We became Elephant. The second album, *Caught Stuck Behind*, was professionally manufactured at a cassette processing plant in Tennessee. The package included a full colour insert, liner notes, and a band photo. It cost a fair amount, but it was worth it. We had a release party at a local club, followed by a string of shows through southwestern Ontario in the fall of 1992. Many school days began with me passed out in a study carrel in the school library during period one (reeking of the bar and the road, having arrived home from a show in Hamilton, Guelph, or Kingston as my dad was getting up to make his oatmeal), and me signing a copy of *Caught Stuck Behind* from my seat in period two History.

○ ○ ○

You would think that being in a band would have made me a lightning rod for the romantic attentions of our female fans, but while the other members of the band may have been getting some action, it was *not* true for me. There was one exception, though, and that exception is the reason for this whole foray into my musical past.

In March 1992, I came to be walking across the basketball court in the St. Anne High School gym. I was there to see Jeff Mingay, singer and guitar player for the band Ghrl, play in one of his final high-school basketball games. He went to a different high school out in Tecumseh, but through our musical connection, we had become close friends.

When the game was over, I crossed the court to congratulate him and tell him where to meet up for drinks. As the oft-repeated family story goes, I was spotted from the stands by a St. Anne student, who asked her friends "Who's that guy talking to Jeff Mingay?" And, as she tells it today, her friends excitedly told her that *that* was Bob Stewart, the lead singer of Elephant.

That young woman's name was Jennifer Daley. She showed up very early for one of our shows a few nights later at the Coach & Horses. She was of course very pretty and sweet and chatty, and she didn't seem to mind at all that I was drinking alone in the bar when she found me. Apparently, I was very bad at reading the signs she was sending out. Although she came to subsequent Elephant shows and started hanging out at the Coach and other downtown venues to see other bands, and we ended up at more than a few of the same parties (she even drove me to a bonfire out in the county with a gaggle of her girlfriends, where I passed out in a soy field), we did not officially become a couple for over a year.

"Can I write letters to you?" she asked one night at the end of the summer of 1993. She was heading back to the University of Guelph, 300 kilometres northeast of Windsor, to begin the second year of her undergrad. I was about to begin an English and Creative Writing degree at the University of Windsor — I had elected to stay in town and pursue Elephant's destiny and the reading lists and writing workshops that I hoped would turn me into a novelist. Writing letters to a pretty girl in another town seemed like a great way to hone my writing chops.

During the first six weeks of that fall semester, we probably averaged about four letters to each other per week. Jennifer would keep me abreast of the goings-on in Guelph, all the crazy things she and the ladies would get up to in the pub and in residence and what books had been assigned in her second year English and French courses. I would fill her in on the latest Elephant gossip or song writing binges, hilarious anecdotes from parties, how strange I found my introductory creative writing workshops.

Needless to say, when Jennifer came home for Thanksgiving weekend in October, we had amassed quite a correspondence and, whether I knew it or not, were primed for romance. She called me Thanksgiving Sunday and said, "A bunch of us are going out for coffee after Thanksgiving dinner. I can pick you up."

There ended up being just four other people, including Jennifer. Maybe it was the tryptophan in the turkey, but the coffee wasn't working, and it wasn't really a drinking crowd, so the night seemed to wind down quickly. Jennifer's plan was to drop her other friends off first and then drive me home. Somehow, we ended up in a woodlot out in the county, and then we decided to check out a giant mound of dirt piled up in the middle of a housing development. It was dark, it was October, and when we lay down on the compacted cold earth on the side of the hill, we could see a surprising number of stars. We kissed for the first time.

When she returned to university, our correspondence continued with renewed vigour and new depths of intimacy. There were revelations: I learned Jennifer had been born in Toronto but moved to Montreal then Halifax, relocating as her father pursued his advertising and publishing career; that she had been seriously contemplating entering a convent, becoming someone known as Sister Philippa, before her father took an executive position with Chrysler Canada. Jennifer decided to follow the family to Windsor, enrolling in tenth grade at St. Anne High School and leaving Sacred Heart School in Halifax behind. Admittedly, this sudden deep dive into Catholicism caught me off guard. I knew, of course, that she had attended Catholic school, but I had always assumed that that was something young people were forced to do by their parents; that it couldn't possibly be a rational choice someone made. *Was it cause for concern? Was it going to become an issue and derail our young relationship?*

I decided that I needed to get Jennifer up to speed on my atheism, which could more truthfully be called a bunch of confused opinions and biases I held against anything that had to do with the idea of God, or faith, or church — a grudge I took on as a six-year-old when I found out, partially through my mom being honest with me and partially through eavesdropping, that my maternal grandparents, staunch members of the Salvation Army, had been opposed to my mother marrying my father because although he was Scottish by name, his people were unbaptized French-Canadians who lived amongst First Nations People in the woods of Quebec.

As a child, I found this slight against my parents infuriating; I believed that it had something to do with God. The fact that my dad was being judged for it infuriated me even more. And in that moment, in my naïveté, my atheism was born, and I carried it before me for many years, like my own personal godless Arc of the Covenant. The only person who knew about the origins of this cross I'd been bearing for the last thirteen years was me.

Now, I was sharing it with a girl I was in love with to — *strangely* — bare more of my soul to her and in a subtle effort to disabuse her of her faith. Jennifer said she understood how faith can be a difficult thing for some people to connect with and that she understood some of my (very rote) criticisms, but otherwise, she did not take the bait. And her decision to not engage me on the subject of faith made me think I had the upper hand — that I held the intellectually superior high ground — and I operated under this delusion for years.

Along with exchanging letters, we also began talking on the phone at night, when the long-distance rates went down, as there was some news too urgent for the Victorian pace of the mail. "Elephant's been nominated for a Jammy," I told her one night, lying on my little captain's bed in my bedroom in my parents' home, reading from the nomination letter we had received at our corporate address (Sean's dad's dental office had become the de facto headquarters of our music publishing company, Slack Music). The Jammies were

CJAM's annual local music awards, and the awards ceremony provided a showcase for Windsor bands — and was obviously a huge party. *Caught Stuck Behind* had charted high at CJAM, as well as at some other college radio stations across the country. I wasn't sure if the ceremony (and the party) was the kind of thing I should invite Jennifer down for. She would have to take the train from Guelph. "We're playing a short, five-song set, and maybe we will win an award, too. So, I don't know if you want to —"

"I'll buy my ticket tomorrow," she said.

On November 16, I walked the few hundred metres from Neitherworld Studio to the VIA station to greet Jen's evening train coming in. She was surprised to see me, and a bit embarrassed, I think, as her mother was there to pick her up and take her home to see her family and have supper. It was the first time I met the woman who would become my mother-in-law. I'm not sure if I passed muster in my flight jacket and plaid flannel, but I got a chaste little hug from Jennifer in the VIA station concourse before she was hustled into the waiting car with a promise that she would see me at Changez by Nite — the goth-tinged dance and rock bar where the Jammies were being held — in a few hours. I walked back to the studio in a goofy-grinned daze, buoyed by the certainty that we were going to win the award.

And we did. Elephant won the 1993 Jammy Award for Best Local Band. Our set was tight, energetic, and loud, just the way we liked it. And Jennifer was there to see it, sitting with all the other band girlfriends back by the soundboard. When we were done our set, I took her by the hand and, emboldened by the night's success, said "Let's go for a walk."

We slipped out the stage door and found ourselves in the alley that ran along the west side of the club. It was a rainy night, and we walked north up the alley. I wasn't quite sure where we were going, but we stopped at around the same time and kissed.

"I think I want to go out with you," I said.

"I think I want to say yes."

And now we were a couple. *Officially.* Our declaration was made standing in an alley in what is, to this day, one of the sleaziest, most crime-addled parts of the city. But we were happy.

And I was still happy when we returned to Changez. The DJ sets were underway and the dancefloor was hopping; the party was still in full swing. Of course, I had a drink to celebrate. And several more.

For the next three years, Jennifer and I burned up the phone lines — the postal system and the rail lines smouldered, too — and our relationship flourished despite the 300 kilometres between us. We met each other's parents, spent time at each other's family homes during summers and holidays — we *became* family quickly, and my trips to visit Jennifer in Guelph increased in frequency and duration. We would spend the days in bed or in bookstores and cafes. And we loved to eat — whether we were trying new restaurants, old favourites, or working in the kitchen together, food was a big part of the relationship.

But not booze. Although she drank with me, Jennifer was not much of a drinker, and her attempts to keep up with the crowd I drank with were ill-fated. She soon developed more of a taste for *not getting sick.* My drinking continued, unfettered. If anything, it increased in volume. This wasn't just the result of alcoholism's steady progression; it happened because I was secure and loved, and because I was willing to use those things as a shield against criticism and judgment — two of the things every alcoholic fears the most.

Small weekend-long tours and endless writing and rehearsal sessions in the Neitherworld resulted in a ton of new, sonically adventurous material for Elephant (inventive guitar tunings, difficult beats, more challenging and bizarre subject matter). We needed to record the new stuff; it was time to get back into the studio.

Compact disc technology was now within reach financially, and we were one of the first Windsor bands to release material on a CD. With Andrew working the board and friends from other bands sitting in on additional guitars, synths, and backing vocals, we crafted *You My Pacifier* through the spring and summer of 1994 and launched it to a fair amount of media buzz in the fall.

Soon after, the inevitable personal politics and artistic differences that haunt every creative partnership boiled over and led to Pat's departure from the band. It could have been a fatal blow, but Andrew had been piloting our ship for so long, he slid right into the lineup. He knew all the songs and brought along a slew of fresh new ideas. Material for a fourth recording was starting to percolate, and when Jennifer arrived home from Guelph in May 1995, Elephant was just getting ready to hit the road for a string of shows that stretched through the summer. I was being pulled in two directions. I was excited to be on the road, performing and partying with the band, and desperate to stay home and read John Irving novels — Jennifer introduced me to them — in the sun next to her parents' pool in St. Clair Beach.

"Don't be silly," she told me. "You guys have been working toward this for so long. Just be safe, and when you get home, I will be here. Besides, I will be working for my dad most days."

"I worry sometimes that you'll get sick of this," I said, not really knowing what I meant by "*this.*"

She laughed and reassured me I was being silly and mopey. "I'm not going anywhere," she said. "And neither are you. You're just going to be in other places knocking them dead."

She was right about our relationship, of course, but wrong about the tour. Although some of the nights were memorable, others were forgettable, or flat out *regrettable* — the road was totally unpredictable. Poor turnouts in the big cities (Toronto, Hamilton, Ottawa), freaky turnouts in the smaller towns (Sarnia, Kingston, and St.

Mary's), spending *way more* money than we were bringing in plagued the tour.

By the time that summer wound down and the tour was behind us, we were physically exhausted, financially broken, and a little bit sick of each other. We arrived back in Windsor after what was supposed to have been the best summer of our lives with our tails between our legs and a bad taste in our collective mouths. *Had I missed Jennifer too much and consequently painted everything with a negative brush? What had gone wrong? Why had we played to a nearly empty room in London? Was the new material not as good as the old? Where had all the money gone?*

In the wake of that summer, we almost moved to Toronto — the whole band, all our girlfriends, including Jennifer. The thinking was it would be cheaper to tour if we were based in the centre of the Canadian music scene. We were making plans, thinking about housing and practice space and jobs … *and then we just didn't.* Undergraduate degrees and careers hung in the balance, and in the end, the pressure those things exerted on our lives coupled, I think, with the toll taken by life on the road (not to mention the fact that we were not exactly getting rich or famous) put the kibosh on the move.

School started. There was a tearful goodbye with Jennifer as she headed back up to Guelph for the final year of her undergrad, and I threw myself into my third year of English at Windsor with a new avidity that in hindsight was likely driven by the need to make a clean break with what had, for seven years, been a big part of my life. When John called me a few weeks later to get a rehearsal schedule hashed out, my response was, "I think I'm done." At twenty-one years old, I didn't have it in me anymore. I really loved the good times, but I did not want to weather the bad times. My ego couldn't take it. And I think, on some level, Sean, John, and Andrew felt the same way. There was very little discussion and zero acrimony.

○   ○   ○

It was during this time that the pounds really started to pile up. I had traded in the dubious, indolent life of an indie rock musician for the wholly sedentary, louche life of reading and writing into the wee hours (on the nights when I wasn't out getting wasted and smoking entire packs of cigarettes with my friends).

"Bobby, you're putting on a lot of weight," said my dad one day, doing as bad a job of concealing his disappointment as I was doing concealing my girth in clothes that a year earlier had fit me just fine.

"Thanks," I said, staring deep into the fridge, knowing he was saying it out of love and concern, but still mortified, and needing to eat all the more because of it.

"Do you have to drink every time you go out with your friends?" my mom asked when I rose after noon one day after coming home near dawn and struggling for several minutes to get my key in the lock, a cacophony that sounded like a bear trying to claw through the oak in the dead of night.

"I don't," was my idiotic reply, and, where seconds before the thought of eating would have brought my gorge into the back of my throat, I now opened the fridge to bury my shame and guilt in food.

"Does Jen say anything to you about it?" my mom asked.

"About going out with my friends?"

"No, about your drinking."

"No, just you."

And that was true. Jennifer had completed her degree in Guelph and moved home to begin a degree in education at Windsor. We saw each other almost every day. If we spent part of the evening together — dinner, a movie, shopping, watching TV, reading together, snuggling … all those normal, nice things that young couples do — the evening would more often than not end with me kissing her goodnight when she dropped me off at my parents' house, making a few quick phone calls, and then heading out to wherever the drinking was happening. And on the nights she was out with me, she would often be paying for the drinks that my mother seemed to be implying would eventually divide us. She would clean me up when, on occasion, as every drunk does, I puked all over a bathroom or bedroom. She would hold the cold cloth to my head and the straw to my lips as I slept off a brutal hangover in her little wooden bed, in her bedroom, in her parents' home.

She never said anything about my drinking.

Somehow, my marks were incredible. Papers I was writing on Thomas Hardy, Tim O'Brien, Nathanael West, Walter Benjamin, Orson Welles, and Thomas Nagel were coming back with A+s on them. I was encouraged to apply for grad school, and was accepted everywhere I applied, including Windsor. But when the acceptance came in from McGill University in Montreal ...

"You have to go," Jennifer said, tears distorting her blue eyes. "I will miss you, and it will be hard, but you were here the whole time I was in Guelph. We can do it. And you will be home for Thanksgiving and Christmas and summer, and I will come visit you whenever I can."

She was right. I was scared of leaving home and of leaving her behind. Being on a band tour for weeks at a time with your three best friends was not the same as moving to a city in a different province, where they spoke a different language. My address would change. My phone number would change. I would have to pay for everything, including my right to be at that address. But booze was cheap in Montreal, and you could drink on the streets if you kept it in a paper bag.

CHAPTER TWO

LA CONSOMMATION

MY DAD WONDERED, perhaps, if the admissions office at the oldest and arguably most prestigious university in Canada had made some kind of mistake. Maybe I didn't present as what he thought of as *grad school material* when I was stumbling in the door just before dawn, tripping up the stairs, and knocking things over in my bedroom while trying to find the light switch; or on the more than one time he, upon waking to get ready for work with his half-grapefruit and bowl of oatmeal, found me passed out in a chair in front of the TV in my underwear with a half-eaten sandwich on my bare chest, but in my mind, I was *literary material*. I hadn't written a story yet, but I liked the idea of being a writer, and Montreal seemed like just the place to do that.

By the time I arrived in Montreal to begin my M.A. at McGill in the late summer of 1997, I probably weighed 260 pounds. Jennifer and I drove up together in her purple Dodge Neon so I could take possession of my apartment on Durocher Street in

Milton Park — the neighbourhood immediately east of the campus, affectionately and more commonly known as the McGill Ghetto. My parents arrived a couple of days later with a trailer of furniture and all my books and music and headed back to Windsor after getting me settled in and making sure my fridge and cupboards were packed with food. Jennifer stayed for a few extra days but had to race back to Windsor on Labour Day in order to be in front of a classroom of children on the Tuesday — her first official day as a teacher.

"You're going to do great," I told her as we stood hugging in the morning sun in front of my apartment.

"*You're* going to do great," she said, never tiring of these tearful goodbyes. "Write lots. And call lots. And work on your stories."

"That's why I'm here," I said, wiping tears away with the back of my wrist.

"I'll see you in six weeks," she said. "At Thanksgiving." And with that she got into her little purple car. "I love you," she said out the window, and I watched as she headed south on Durocher, signalled right, and merged with traffic on Sherbrooke, bound for the highway, the provincial border, and the thousand-kilometre drive home.

I stood there crying on the sidewalk for a bit. My heart hurt. My throat burned from upset. A bell jingled, and a man exited the door of the street-level storefront of the high-rise Expo-era apartment building next door to my First World War–era brownstone. I composed myself, walked into the depanneur, bought a case of beer, a pack of cigarettes, and two bags of chips, and returned to my apartment. If I was going to miss Jennifer this much, I was going to miss her with style.

Some people pick up and move cities as a way to escape bad habits and lower companions. But when I went to Montreal, my drinking, my behaviour, and my personality unfortunately followed.

Changing locales turned out to be no cure at all, especially when I had no intention of even tapering back on my lifestyle. No. The validation given by my acceptance into grad school was great; the opportunity to work on my writing made it feel like it was finally about to happen — but I arrived in Montreal to actively pursue my drinking and to find new people to drink with.

As a result of my dedication to my craft, my alcoholism exploded in Montreal, as did every other tendency to overindulge. Sure, you could bring your own booze to restaurants, and it was true, you could walk down the street with an open container as long as you had a paper bag over it, but those things were trivialities compared to the fact that, for the first time in my life, I was living on my own. I didn't have to worry about disappointing my parents. I could eat, smoke, and drink whenever I wanted. Within a week, I had a solid weed connection. I could wake up and make steak and eggs and polish off the red wine from the night before, music cranked, a joint burning between my lips.

A couple of days into classes, I was standing on the terrace at the McLennan Library during a break in the mandatory Bibliography and Research Methods course each new M.A. student is subjected to, smoking a cigarette as the campus and city buzzed around me. I made eye contact with a guy I recognized from the class. He was wiry and had dirty-blond hair pulled back in a short ponytail, crooked glasses, and a goofy grin. I can't remember how the conversation went exactly, but it was something like this:

Me: You're in Suvin's practicum, right?

Him: Yeah. I like R.E.M.

Me: Wanna drink in my apartment after this? I have all their albums.

Him: Yes.

Michael Epp — Saskatchewan Mennonite, Flann O'Brien scholar, R.E.M. fan. We were inseparable for the next two years.

Rumours actually circulated about our relationship in our contentious and catty little M.A. cohort, which we found very funny. But we were just two guys who liked to get drunk and high, listen to music, talk books, watch hockey, and check out flicks at Cinema du Parc, the amazing rep cinema situated just blocks from the McGill Ghetto.

Nights on the town often ended back at my apartment, and whether there was a crowd or just me and Mike drunk and stoned out of our minds, whole pizzas and four-for-the-price-of-three poutines were ordered with such regularity the guy who answered the phone at Mama's Restaurant didn't even need to hear a voice or an address to know what was being ordered and where it was headed.

Despite all the fun I was having, McGill ended up not being a good fit for me academically. My work on Don DeLillo and David Foster Wallace and expressionism in the films of David Lynch found little traction with the faculty or my peers. This made it a lot easier for me to lose interest in being a literary scholar at McGill and become more enamoured with being a writer in Montreal. For the first time in my life, I was free to engage in the reckless indolence that seemed crucial to getting any writing done — walking stoned from cafe to cafe during the day, reading Auster, Pynchon, Donald Barthelme, and Cormac McCarthy while whiling away the hours between the serious drinking.

Despite the indolence, I was actually getting some writing done, working on the stories I promised Jennifer I would work on. Oddly enough, the story that was getting most of my attention, now that I was a writer in Montreal, was a story set back home in Windsor, on the street I'd grown up on — Iroquois Street — where my parents still lived. Set during a residential street replacement project, the story is about the dissolution of a marriage told from the perspective of a young writer who, working from home all day during the road construction, observes the infidelities of his neighbours and the tragic events that lead-up to a family pet being tumble-dried to death. The story was called "There is No Brown Glass Forest"; looking back, it's pretty clear the story is about alcoholism. Other people's alcoholism but alcoholism, nonetheless.

I had never been much for that old creative writing workshop chestnut, "Write what you know!" but I did like the idea of taking things I saw or heard — things I had observed from my boyhood bedroom window, things like a bikini-clad neighbour, her skin tanned to an unholy shade of catcher's-mitt brown, inviting a veritable conga line of road crew workers into her home for drinks and who knew what other delights, while her husband was at work — and sharpening them through the lens of fiction.

The social lubricant of booze and the expansive properties of marijuana seemed to aid me at every turn in my initial immersion in the writing life. Suddenly, story ideas were presenting themselves to me in virtually every conversation I had in a bar — tall tales, scandalous anecdotes, overheard dialogue. I was constantly running off to the washroom to jot things down in the notebook I began to carry with me.

I found material I could exploit everywhere: the self-effacing story of a friend walking in on a caterer changing into her livery at a wedding and becoming obsessed with her; my memory of a strange community of houseboats along the Detroit River where my father was bitten by a black widow spider the summer I worked for his appliance and furniture delivery business; the collected (and fictionalized) phone conversations of a depressed, drunken English professor who would call his former students at night and cry into the phone in a way that definitely got more creepy and sad as the story progressed; the visceral and heroic story of some local men — doctors, dentists, lawyers (all the fathers of friends of mine) — who saved a young girl from a vicious dog attack and then took it upon themselves to seek revenge on the dogs …

There was no shortage of ideas; my notebooks provided tangible proof of the feverish state of my imagination as I cranked out stories. Some of these I read at open mics and parties around Montreal. Eventually, I opened up a *Writer's Market* catalogue (in the pre-internet days, this telephone book–sized tome provided a listing of all the publishers and journals accepting work from writers), and hit the post office with my manuscripts, a list of prospective journals and literary magazines, and self-addressed stamped envelopes for their replies.

I often received no reply from the small journals and literary zines, as is common. Many of my stories and my self-addressed stamped envelopes simply disappeared into the slush pile in some overworked grad student cubicle, never reaching their destination at all. But some of those stories did find their way to an editor's desk, and the replies that came back to my steel mailbox in the foyer of my Durocher Street apartment were all form rejection letters, thanking me for the opportunity to read my work and wishing me luck in my future endeavours.

It was always a disappointment, but I was having too much fun to quit. Sadly, I found that what I enjoyed, more than writing, was *being a writer*. The first, I was learning, was work; the other was a lifestyle. Even if you weren't a published writer, you could live like a writer. And I was finding I had a natural inclination to do just that.

Few things gave me more pleasure during those cold Montreal winters than returning to my apartment after a night along Saint Laurent Boulevard — maybe with a few smoked meats from The Main Deli in a greasy paper sack — turning on some music, lighting a joint, pouring a tumbler of Scotch, and writing until the sun came up.

Stan, who ran the depanneur under the high-rise next door, got used to seeing me standing out on the fire escape in my plaid robe when he would arrive, pre-dawn, to open the shop. I would waggle a few fingers on one hand and tap my lips with two fingers of the other. He would nod and disappear into the store. When he came back out, he would stand on the concrete beneath the fire escape and toss king cans of beer and packs of smokes up to me. I would settle up with him later in the evening when I went in to buy the full case I needed to get through the night. He was cool with the arrangement and so was I. He knew where I lived, and he knew I was going to be coming back for more. I saw him nearly every day for nearly two years, and our conversations never moved beyond the Habs and the particulars of our transactions.

A pattern was forming in Montreal's long, dark winters, and it only added to the list of things that were not good for me.

"I feel like a vampire," I said to Jennifer on the phone one night. "My life is taking place totally in the nighttime. I go out at night, I come home and write until morning, I go to bed, I wake up and it's dark again. I eat breakfast at five thirty at night, and it starts all over. I can't remember the last time I was up during the day."

"Well, maybe you just need to change the pattern," she said. "Go to bed when you hang up the phone, get up in the morning and make sure you get outside for a bit. Go for a walk, go to the library — are you crying?"

I was crying. I told her it was because I missed her, and I probably *did* just need some sunshine, but I didn't tell her that something had happened the night before. On a rare night where I hadn't left my apartment to meet up with Mike and select drinking associates, I'd sat down on the couch with a bowl of cereal to watch television and inexplicably burst into tears. Unable to stop, I started feeling numbness in my left arm and jaw. I started trying to monitor my heart rate and my breathing.

I'd thought about calling Mike — he lived a block away, but he was probably out; besides, I didn't want to come off as a blubbering mess. I was supposed to be cool. I thought about calling my parents. My mom was a nurse and would know what to do, but they were a thousand kilometres away, and I didn't want to scare them: their adult son calling just before midnight, sobbing into the phone. And of course, I thought about calling Jennifer, who was now my fiancée (I'd asked her to marry me a few months earlier while home for Christmas), but I didn't want her to know that things weren't going well. She was proud of me. She had a classroom full of kids to teach in the morning and didn't need to be preoccupied with whatever embarrassing state I had worked myself into. Of course, I wasn't really cognizant of how depressed I was. Treating depression with a depressant was certainly not doing my spirits any favours. I found myself sleeping off the hangovers, sleeping through the darkest blues during the day to get to the part when I could drink like a gentleman and have huge panic attacks at night.

But the sound of her soft, reassuring voice giving solid, practical advice resulted in me weeping into the handset. Jennifer calmed me down and soothed me with that mix of sympathy and unflinching realism that works on people like me. "You're not dying," she told me, when I told her that I was, in fact, afraid that I was dying. "You just need to do something different."

I found myself in the walk-in closet in my apartment's front hall, pulling jackets off the hooks that lined the wall until I found what I was looking for: a pair of swimming goggles. And then, a few hooks later, the Speedo bathing suit and cap, last worn during my days on my high-school swim team. Somehow, these two items had made the move to Montreal. Like my Aunt Shirley who, as a toddler during the Great Depression, was found sitting in the garden filling her mouth with rocks because she was anemic, I was compelled by instinct — and by Jennifer's instruction to *change the pattern* — to do something.

I knew that that ancient building around the corner on Sherbrooke housed McGill's Garfield-Weston Pool (known around campus as the "Old Pool") — all terrazzo and tile and the heavy miasma of chlorine. As it turned out, as a card-carrying McGill grad student, I could swim there for free. There were hours set aside every morning for lap swimming. I figured maybe I could stem the tide of some of my late-night pizza and poutine crushing and started walking to the Old Pool in the early mornings, not bothering to bring anything with me other than the essentials. They had towel service!

I felt extremely self-conscious in the few frantic moments before I lowered myself into the pool after gingerly crossing the deadly wet terrazzo of the pool deck, exposed in my corpulence like a gluttonous fawn crossing an open field. But despite my ballooning weight, I was still a strong swimmer. I enjoyed using the old-fashioned analogue lap clock on the wall to time my lengths, and even more, I enjoyed how I felt when I was done. I would return to my apartment a bit tired but pleasantly loose and refreshed and, after a coffee and a mammoth breakfast, ready to take on the day.

You'd think adding an hour of swimming every morning to my daily routine would have made me a paragon of health in a student ghetto, but aside from the swimming, I changed absolutely nothing about the way I was living. Consequently, though my first serious bout of depression may have lifted ever so slightly, nothing else about my life changed.

And then one Montreal winter morning, I was waiting to cross University Street (now Robert-Bourassa Boulevard) at Sherbrooke when a group of students sidled up next to me waiting for the light to change so we could clamber over the boot print–pocked hummock of gravel-encrusted snow that was plowed like a fortification around every street corner in the city from November to March. Someone said, "Hey man, are you okay?" and I realized they were talking to me. I turned to see a guy, bundled up against the tooth-shattering temperatures, looking me up and down with concern as

I stood there in a cloud of steam. The people he was with were also giving me the serious side-eye.

"I was just swimming laps," I said, gesturing behind them to the low, nineteenth-century swimming pavilion that housed the Old Pool.

"Yeah, but man, it's cold out here!" he said, incredulous. "There's steam coming off you. There is ice on your head!"

I raised my bare hand to my head and felt the sharp scaling of ice forming over a slippery, smooth surface. *He was right.* And this is how I found myself walking around the frozen streets of Montreal in that same thin, plaid robe Stan saw flapping like a pennant on the fire escape in the mornings, my bare feet tucked into moccasin-style slippers, a bathing cap with goggles mounted up on my forehead, steam rising from every part of me, including the dripping-wet Speedo, which is all I wore beneath the robe.

"I just live here in the Ghetto," I offered, as if people didn't freeze to death on the streets, and when the light turned green, over the treacherous mound of snow I went, robe flapping around my bare ankles. But I was suddenly aware of the ridiculous futility of my swimming regimen and how lunatic I looked shuffling through the frigid metropolis in slippers and a robe, a rind of ice forming on my bathing cap. Although I had been aware that this was how I was setting out from my apartment under cover of the early morning darkness, I had lost sight of something essential, something important that I couldn't quite put my finger on. It bothered me that I didn't know what it was, but I knew this for certain: *something was wrong with me.*

Minutes later, I stopped in to see Stan at the dep. My regular morning swims had curtailed (somewhat) our early-morning fire escape routine but had somehow failed to take so much as a few pounds off my body. No one was paying me any compliments, and my flip turn was as bad as it had been when the Speedo had actually fit me in high school. I grabbed a couple of king cans, a pack of smokes, and a box of cereal that I would eat over the next few hours before sleeping through the rest of the day, until people started making plans of where we were going to drink that evening.

And rather than simply making a concession to seasonally appropriate clothing and using a change-room locker to store my street clothes while swimming, I just stopped making the trip to the Old Pool altogether. That brief interaction on the corner marked the end of my brief flirtation with swimming. And by the time the weather was nice enough to make my Old Pool–look at least seasonally acceptable, I was getting ready to move back to Windsor.

○ ○ ○

I returned to Windsor in May 1999, an emotionally unstable and beaten-down drunk with a Master's degree and a clutch of rejection letters. My weight had breached the three-hundred-pound threshold and I was, once again, living in my parents' home. My wedding day was twelve months away.

I wasn't fitting into my clothes very well, but I slid very easily back into old routines with old friends, hitting all the old haunts. I told everyone I was done with academia because I was sick of the pretentious people and posturing — that was true — but failing to add that I was sick of them because I was emotionally unstable and so committed to being a drinker-about-town that I couldn't focus on the rigours of academic research and writing.

I landed a salaried job as the editor of a local sports newspaper, but that went bankrupt within four months. I stumbled on, landing a brief string of jobs not exactly in keeping with how I envisioned my post–Master's degree career trajectory but wholly befitting what I was capable of at the time. The first was working the midnight shift at the bakery that supplied doughnuts and other pastries to the various Tim Hortons in the city. Jennifer and my parents were thrilled that I had found "steady work" and were vocally disappointed when I quit via phone call the morning after my first disastrous single-handed shift, in which I shorted the city by several hundred doughnuts.

A few days later, over pints, I was talked into signing on with a landscaping crew run by some British soccer hooligans I'd met at a bar. (Since the work was weather-dependent, many days degenerated into a tour of local watering holes.) "There's nothing wrong with working with your hands," Jennifer said as I sat staring blankly into the middle-distance, stunned by the realization that the kind of work I had gone to grad school to avoid doing had become the only work that was available to me.

Naturally, I didn't realize how fortunate I was to be engaged to a person who was still willing to accept me as I was, when I was unwilling to accept anything about my status and equally unwilling to take any reasonable action to change. Two years into her career as an elementary school teacher, Jennifer had saved enough money to buy us a house — a two-storey, 1911-vintage, double-brick and original-hardwood affair on Moy Avenue in Walkerville. It was a place we could call our own with a possession date a few weeks before our wedding.

One of the ways I found to repay her love and kindness was by constantly attacking her faith. I felt the need to tell her that her job teaching in the Catholic school system was tantamount to brainwashing children. Of course, I conveniently ignored the fact that this job was keeping a roof over my head, buying enough food for me to eat myself into gastric distress nearly every night when I got home from the bars. Not mentioned either was fact that the twenty or so drinks I consumed each night were being paid for, by and large, out of Jennifer's single income. My rantings on the subject of her faith and profession were met with silence. I was pleased to note that over time Jennifer's attendance at her church waned and that the rosary and crucifix she had mounted on the wall above her night table simply disappeared. I didn't gloat, but I did consider myself victorious on the matter of faith in our relationship.

About a week after signing the mortgage papers, I got in an argument with the owner of the landscaping company, who'd left me at a job site with a trailer of lawn maintenance equipment and no fuel with which to fulfill the contract. I quit on the spot and walked home to my parents' house, pleased with myself for not sullying the new home Jennifer and I would be moving into in a matter of days by dragging a job I felt was beneath me across the threshold on muddied work boots.

I washed the stench of not even a month of landscaping work from my body (nothing about the hard labour having made a dent in my mounting obesity), made a pot of coffee, and sat down with the newspaper. There was an ad: the *Windsor Star* newsroom was looking for a reporter/photographer to cover the county beat. "That is my new job," I said aloud, sitting in my parents' sun-drenched living room that March afternoon.

I immediately sent in my resume, complete with clippings from my tenure at the short-lived sports newspaper. Later that evening, once she got home from her day in the classroom, I called Jennifer at her parents' house. "I quit the landscaping job today," I said. "But there's good news —"

"We move into our house in a couple of weeks, and we are getting married in two months and you quit another job?!" She was furious. "I just don't understand you. Why would you quit your job at a time like this?"

"Those guys were jerks," I said. "Besides — this is what I was going to tell you before you cut me off — I applied for a job at the *Windsor Star*. They're looking for a reporter and a photographer to cover the county."

"You had better hope this works," she said quietly, dubiously. "I don't know what we'll do if you don't have a job."

"Don't worry," I said. "I'm going to get this job."

And I did. I got the job. I started at the *Windsor Star* on Easter weekend, 2000, a week after we moved into the house. A month later Jennifer and I were married. On the surface, it appeared as if things were looking up. All the trappings of wedded domestic bliss were in place. But none of these positive changes in my life served to quell my appetites.

Jennifer made an effort to bring only healthy foods into the house, avoiding snack foods and things she knew I was powerless over — a list that by rights should have included things like cheese, meat, and bread — but my appetites were out of control. I would eat supper at home then I would often eat another full meal of bar food, pulled hot from the grease fryer a couple hours later, before grabbing some street meat or a couple of Whoppers on the way home at 2:00 a.m. This was a typical weekday night, aided and abetted by the permissive workplace culture of the newspaper and a steady paycheque.

◦ ◦ ◦

Nights running up a tab at the Press Club and eating in my car in strip-mall parking lots took their toll on my mornings. As permissive as the *Star*'s newsroom culture was, you were expected to be at your desk by 10:00 a.m., and it was becoming a problem. Even if I got downtown with time to spare, finding parking necessitated making a miserable circuit around the old *Star* building at Ferry and Pitt. Nearby parking garages either required a big cash outlay up front for a monthly parking pass, or they chipped away at your pocket money, one day at a time. I wanted that money to drink with, and metered parking required a literally breathtaking amount of running back and forth to your vehicle with change every two hours to avoid a ticket.

One morning early in my *Star* tenure, I noticed the metered spots right outside the paper's stately front entrance were often empty when I was driving around, gaseous and hungover, looking for a spot with ever increasing urgency as the clock ticked down toward 10:00 a.m. If I was going to have to make a couple of trips to deposit coins in the meter that morning, so be it. I would move the car at lunch.

I pulled into a spot, hauled my camera bag out of the back seat, and headed toward the newspaper's grand facade. Because of the church-and-state separation of editorial and sales staff, journalists were not supposed to use the front door, nor travel through the ground-level administrative and sales floor of the building. All newsroom staff had a special swipe card that gave them access, through a discreet door along Pitt Street, which led directly to an elevator to the third floor. But I was in no shape to make the long walk around the side of the building that day. I was nauseous and already sweating through my shirt. I looked up and down the street to make sure there were no senior newsroom people about and entered through the chiselled marble archway into the newspaper's main lobby.

Carrying myself like a man who had spent a career walking through that very door and across that polished lobby, I headed up the grand staircase, navigated some service stairwells, and was sitting at my desk in the third-floor newsroom, dyspeptic but present, perusing that day's paper with minutes to spare. I got busy, skipped lunch because of my queasy stomach, and it wasn't until late in the afternoon I remembered my car sitting out front at the parking meter. I retraced what I assumed was my personal, secret route back to the front door. I expected to see the windshield of my salsa-red Dodge Neon papered with tickets, but there it sat, fine-free.

The next day, hungover and running late once again, I decided to push my luck. And the day after that. One of the half-dozen spots in front of the building always seemed available, and city parking enforcement seemed to relax their stranglehold on downtown along this stretch of Ferry Street. But while I was celebrating going undetected at the parking meter, I had forgotten about the strict observance of segregation that was to be maintained between editorial and sales for the sake of the paper's journalistic integrity. And in that forgetting, I, myself, had been *observed*.

A couple of weeks into my verboten door-using ways, I was entering the building, weighed down with camera equipment and notebooks, a take-out coffee and a couple of Danishes, trying to manage the compacted chyme and residual blood-alcohol level and vapours of the previous night's vagaries when a voice caught me partially up the grand staircase.

"Excuse me, what is your business at the *Star*?"

I froze. I had known I was getting away with something but really hadn't expected to be called on it. It's not like I was dallying about the ad sales cubicles, hiring out my writing chops for advertorial blowjobs from local vinyl siding companies or realtors. I turned and walked as briskly as possible across the lobby to the old wood-and-glass front counter. "Hi," I said, quietly. "I work in the newsroom; I was just cutting through."

"You work in the newsroom? I've never seen you before. What's your name?" Short and doughy, the woman wore a shapeless flower-print dress; her mouse-grey hair hung limply around her face, which was pinched in an expression of doubt. She was clearly suspicious of my credentials.

"I'm Bob Stewart. I've only been here a few months. I know we're supposed to use the other door, but I was running late and just thought I could pop through —"

"Well, I don't know who you are, and I've been watching you sneaking through the front door and up the stairs for weeks now. What is your business here?"

Behind her, in low wooden carrels, seemingly happy people were going about their administrative and clerical duties in the bright morning sun that shone through the high arched windows. The phone rang; printers and fax machines hummed and chirped their commerce.

"Look, I know. I'm not supposed to use this door, but I'm just cutting through. I've got a really great parking spot out front —"

"Those parking spots are reserved for customers of the *Windsor Star*," she said, venomously. "They are not for reporters or photographers or newsroom people, or whatever it is you do."

"I'm a reporter *and* a photographer," I said. "And I don't see any signs out there saying the spaces are reserved. It's actually metered parking."

"Metered parking reserved for customers of the *Windsor Star*," she barked, slapping the wooden countertop for emphasis.

"Still no signs," I said, skipping merrily up the stairs. "Like I said, I'm running late."

I really wasn't too worried about our exchange. It's not like the publisher or Metro editor had apprehended me under the great lobby chandelier. She was just some busybody gatekeeper from the secretary pool, making life miserable for the journalists. But I was curious to know who, exactly, she was. I asked delicately worded questions around the newsroom — "Hey, what's the name of that haggard shrew who works at the front desk?" — and found out her name was Sandra Voorhees.

I continued to park there several times a week throughout my tenure at the *Star*, and our pitched battle of glares and blown kisses continued over the rich stain of the majestically carved front counter.

The real battle, of course, was being waged inside of me — in my guts, in my liver, and in my head. And it eventually reached a point where, swelled up on boozy pride and feeling wronged because I had been passed over for promotion and adulation after not even two years on the job, I betrayed the confidence of Wayne, the editor-in-chief who took a chance on me because he said he was tired of journalism school grads who could quote chapter and verse from the *CP Style Guide* but didn't know how to tell a story or take a photo, and quit.

I got up from my desk at the end of a long Sunday night shift, quietly left the building, and while sitting at home eating supper, announced, "I'm quitting the *Star.*"

Jennifer put her fork down. "What? *Why?*"

"They don't appreciate me," I said. "I'm tired of watching other reporters pass me by. I haven't told them yet, though." And I picked up the phone and made my young, beleaguered, and strangely resigned bride watch me dial the newsroom — a newsroom I had been working in, seemingly happily, not an hour earlier. I told a night editor who had the misfortune of answering the phone that I was quitting and asked him to tell Wayne for me in the morning. The end.

o o o

Two months later, Jennifer was pregnant. Eager to provide for my family, I took on a number of jobs: marketing coordinator at an arts theatre, customer service rep at a big box bookstore, writer at a marketing agency. I quit all of them before the baby arrived, always for the same reason: my employers didn't understand or appreciate my enormous talents and did not know how to properly stroke my enormous alcoholic ego.

Succor, at least for me, came in the fact that I had embarked on writing a novel — a novel about a young newspaper reporter struggling to write fiction that wasn't inexplicably tied to his journalism career. Of course, the novel, like the short stories that had preceded it, *was* inextricably tied to my journalism career; bits of situations and stories I had covered over the years becoming impastoed upon, woven through, and filigreed around ideas that had been scribbled into a notebook as far back as my years in Montreal. Stories piled up and sank down inside each other — stories about bare-knuckled boxing matches, Indian curry houses, a dentist with a sports car he kept hidden from his family, an international diamond heist happening concurrently with an obscure Russian rock band's tour of eclectic American venues, a woman writing the definitive analytical text on the film *Ferris Bueller's Day Off* ... The hermitic intensity of novel writing allowed me to isolate myself, drunk and stoned, in my home office. It seemed like the next right thing, seeing as how the short stories I was writing were getting roundly rejected and had brought in precisely zero dollars or accolades.

And then, when writing a novel proved too difficult, involved too much toiling in obscurity, resulted in the production of too many individual threads-in-hand for interweaving, I slowly stopped working on my fiction, too. I ended up heading down to Kurley's AC with a book tucked under my arm, a talisman against anyone thinking I was some younger version of the broken-down drunks and ex-jocks who haunted the place.

Yet, despite the fact that I was rarely home at night and despite the fact that our relations were cool — she offered vocal opposition to my extravagant spending and lack of employment (she still had yet to say a word about my drinking) — Jennifer had become pregnant. Our son Nathanael was born in August 2002, and although he was three weeks premature and spent a week in neonatal intensive care with jaundice, those nerve-wracking days of being first-time parents were about the most normal part of a dark period. My life — *our lives*, my drinking — went on like this until February 2003, when I stood bloated and reeking of the previous night's drinks in my doctor's office and he told me I was dying.

I'd shown up in Dr. Sijan's office four days prior with another problem: a vile sinus infection that was making it very difficult for me to enjoy drinking down at Kurley's AC and next to impossible to smoke weed. Brief inspections of my ears, nose, and throat were all he needed to see. He handed me a script for antibiotics and said to me with gravitas, "Robert, what is going on with you?" Dr. Sijan had been my doctor since the day I was born. He had heard all of my health complaints, real and delusional, for years. "I look at you and I see something else is going on."

The alcoholic is as cunning, baffling, and powerful as the disease he suffers from. "Nothing," I said, gesturing to indicate my infected head and bloated face. "It's just this sinus infection. It's killing me."

"Well, I think something else is killing you," he said, suddenly pulling down on my lower eyelids with his confident physician's hands and slapping a blood-pressure cuff on me. I'd been on two different blood pressure medications for several years at this point. Whatever the reading was, it was no surprise. "Robert, I would like to do some blood work," he said in his raspy, Serb-inflected English. "Do you have time to do this today?"

It wasn't really a question. It was his way of saying, "Do this today." He handed me a requisition positively bristling with ticked boxes, and I headed down the hall to the lab, warding off a dread and associated ataxia that I knew went much deeper than my squeamishness around needles. They drained several vials out of me and sent me on my way. Drinking helped me forget that Sijan was on the trail of something, but it didn't stop the phone from ringing four days later. His office nurse told me the doctor needed to see me right away. "It's about your bloodwork," she said. "Can you come in today?"

I remember driving down Walker Road, terrified of what he was going to tell me. *He's going to tell me I have cancer. Or that I have*

MS. Or some dread disease they haven't named yet but will name after me as its very special Patient Zero. Alcoholism simply would not allow me to entertain the possibility that the doctor wanted to talk to me about my drinking.

But that's exactly what he wanted to talk to me about.

"Robert, how much do you drink?" he asked.

I pulled a face, as if I was mining my memory bank in order to give him an accurate count. "I don't know, I maybe have two or three drinks a couple of times a week with friends. Why? Is something wrong?"

"So, maybe six drinks a week?" he asked, providing room for me to multiply that number by something that would make the data on the chart in his hand make sense. He referred to it now. "Robert, you're telling me you drink very moderately, but somehow, at twenty-nine, you have the liver of a man in his sixties who has been drinking heavily all his life. How is that?"

I didn't have an answer for him. Even if I had had one, I probably wouldn't have been able to articulate it for him. The examination room seemed astoundingly bright; sounds became both muffled and too clear. He was looking under my lower lids again, pumping the cuff around my arm. "Robert, if you are telling me you don't drink very much, I need to ask: Do you use intravenous drugs or frequent brothels? The prostitutes?"

"What is wrong with me?" A flat whisper.

"Robert, you are in the early stages of liver failure."

" . . . "

"But if you do not drink, we have a mystery on our hands. What could cause this, Robert? This liver disease in someone who does not use intravenous drugs, or sleep with prostitutes, or drink to excess?" And here he turned his gaze from my blood pressure reading and looked me right in my rheumy, yellow eyes, and said, "Unless, of course, you are not telling me the truth about your drinking."

He was offering me a way out; he was extending to me the ca-duceus of his help.

"I don't know," I heard myself say. "What will happen to me?"

Sijan shrugged. "Liver disease, Robert, is a very tricky thing. You could be dead by Christmas; you could live into your eighties or nineties. But you'll be in a wheelchair and as orange as a carrot, and they'll be cutting off your feet and the tips of your fingers. Either way, we will want to know what's going on. So, we will need to do some tests. I may have to admit you to the hospital for a night or two so we can check your liver function more thoroughly. I will have one of my nurses call you with the details, but in the mean-time, Robert," and here he put his hands on my shoulders, "you cannot drink alcohol. But since you don't really drink, that should not be a problem, right?"

"Right."

"And I should also tell you, Robert, that if we run a bunch of tests and it is clear that this is because of your drinking alcohol then you can either agree to quit drinking or you can find a new doctor," he said. "I will not watch you kill yourself."

Quitting things had become something of a speciality in recent months. But despite Sijan's diagnosis, suspicions, prognosis, and warning, I was not done with drinking. The suggestion that I quit drinking seemed like a gross overreaction. And if his nurse ever called with details about tests and admission to the hospital, I don't remember taking the call, nor do I remember deleting any message. I drank for two more terrified and miserable months before putting down my last drink — a pint of Stella Artois — in the Avalon Front on Ouellette Avenue, on April 11, 2003. I was twenty-nine years old, a husband, a father to a seven-month-old baby boy, a home-owner, an unemployed (and unemployable) professional journalist, and I was no more emotionally mature than that fourteen-year-old boy drinking behind his high school in the freezing cold.

CHAPTER THREE

THE JUMPING-OFF PLACE

THEN THINGS GOT really bad. The next four months of my life were the worst four months of my life. Without alcohol, I was a raw nerve, afraid to leave the house, afraid I was going to hurt myself or someone else.

"Things were better when you were drinking," Jennifer said one evening, sick of my extreme moodiness and moping around the house. And though that may seem harsh, she was right. When I was drinking, I was largely out of the house, operating under alcohol's disastrously temporary mood-elevating effects — the artificial life of the party. Now, I was hanging around the house like a bad smell, sometimes laying in bed for days at a time while Jennifer went off to work and Nathanael, not yet a year old, went to the babysitter we could not afford.

After several weeks of this, a drink started to look too easy and too effective a solution to how I felt. *Where were the benefits of not drinking? Where was the life of alcohol-free bliss and ease I had expected?* I hadn't had a drink in *four months*! Maybe drinking wasn't my problem? Maybe I was broadly misunderstood by my peers and those who loved me? My problems hadn't evaporated like spilled spirits; they'd boiled over like an exploded still. I knew a drink would bring immediate euphoria and ease. Alcohol, like any substance that can be abused, is abused because in the moment, *it works*. Unfailingly. But as tempting as it was, there was some rational part of me that knew I was in this bleak condition because of alcohol.

Lying in bed one day, desperate for relief, the following occurred to me as a single thought: *I can always take a drink. I know what that is like. Or I can just continue to lie here in bed and hide inside the house, hoping my fortunes change. Or I can kill myself. Or, I can just accept the fact that maybe I've been wrong about every aspect of my life to date and do something different …* And in that moment, I was so scared, so beaten down, and so finished with alcohol and the shameful state to which it had brought me that I was no longer afraid of accepting my doctor's diagnosis as the truth.

I broke down and reached out, through the wife of a Kurley's AC drinking associate, for the help of a Twelve Step fellowship. It was like arriving, mercifully, on shore after several years of being adrift on a perilous sea. And I found that by applying some simple principles to my life, one day at a time, I got better. I learned that alcohol, though pernicious to the point of lethality for a drinker of my type, was only a small part of the problem. The larger part was, simply, *who I was* — my character, my thoughts, my actions; the mess I was left with when the obsession with alcohol was removed, mercifully, from my life; the catastrophe of the self.

It's a hell of a thing to be confronted with in the early days of sobriety, but simply *knowing*, and knowing there was a *solution*, was enough hope for me coming down off such a dark precipice. I became less restless, irritable, and discontented. I was able to hold a job and eventually landed back in newspapers as the editor, reporter, and photographer for the *LaSalle Post*, a weekly in LaSalle, Ontario, just southwest of Windsor.

I matured in my behaviour and in my thinking, and as the fog of active alcoholism lifted, my relationships with people improved. Nowhere was this more important than in my relationship with Jennifer, whose steadfastness during even the worst years of my drinking — a steadfastness rooted in her unshakable faith — was instrumental to my recovery.

One night in my early sobriety, I asked Jennifer why, despite all the drinking, the reckless spending, the aloofness, the depression, my fearful atheism … despite all these things, why she stayed. She was sitting in bed reading. She looked up from her magazine to where I stood at the end of the bed, and said, simply, matter-of-factly, "Because I always had faith that you would get better."

She used that word. *Faith.* And in that moment, I knew I needed to grow up and accept that there was something greater than nihilistic chance that had brought me to this moment, something that allowed the wife of a degenerate drinker — a degenerate drinker who openly mocked her faith at every turn — to maintain her faith and have faith in the recovery of the desperately ill man whom she loved.

The atheism borne out of what I saw as the decades-old mistreatment of my parents at the hands of an organized religion; the atheism I had used as a social battering ram to belittle others and make myself feel superior; the atheism that had clearly harmed my relationships with other people by forming what were essentially barriers of religious bigotry — I now saw it for what it was: a form of fear. A fear of confronting my own insignificance and impermanence; a fear of having to revise my personality based on new information; a fear in whose grips I had inflicted deep spiritual harm upon myself by putting up barriers between me and something that, despite my most concerted efforts to think, talk, and act otherwise — and here is the *really* sad and ridiculous part — I had always believed in. Truly, I had never been able to shake my faith.

It was, for many years, the thing I harboured most jealously at my core — not some deep, dark, monstrous secret but a brilliant thing that I did not want to share with anyone. I was so invested in my belief that in university I sought out an undergraduate course in philosophy called The God of Philosophers with the hope that the class would provide me with all the arguments against the existence of God I would need at parties to destroy the faith of believers, burying my fraudulence under further layers of fraudulence. But what I found, to my disgust and dismay, was argument upon argument for the existence of God; arguments that made sense to me, that I could not deny; arguments that actually provided some kind of solace and comfort. All of this threatened the blustery facade of my atheism. So, I did what all good scholars do when confronted with something contrary to their original thesis — I bailed on the class at the drop date and pretended I'd never read any of the material, or heard the open, gentle words of the professor whose admission of his own faith had left me questioning his credentials and embarrassed for him for what was obviously some unresolved simple-mindedness on his part.

Nearly a decade after dropping that course, before the likes of St. Anselm, St. Thomas Aquinas, Blaise Pascal, and William James had the chance to pull aside the curtain of atheism I had hidden myself behind, it was my wife, Jennifer, with the simple, declarative statement she uttered while sitting in bed reading a magazine, who helped me come to believe in a power greater than myself. She helped me to understand that there was a loving, creative force that wanted me to be happy, joyous, and free. I finally came to understand that it was this force that was guiding me toward the things that would ensure I would attain that state — things like fatherhood and a better marriage, which, within the first three years of my sobriety, resulted in the births of our second son, Jonah, in 2005, and our daughter, Thomasin, in 2006.

o o o

Although I was extremely busy balancing the newspaper and fatherhood, I somehow managed to start writing again — *for real this time*. I started to *be* a writer rather than just pretend I was a writer, bragging that I was one at the bar and then passing out drunk in front of my computer on the nights I bothered to try and commit something to the page. But the change was not due to any conscious effort on my part. It just happened one hot afternoon in August 2004, a few days after Nathanael's second birthday.

We had purchased a large inflatable pool we could swim in as a family (there were still just the three of us at the time). When we weren't splashing around with Nathanael, I had taken to reading while sitting in the chest-deep water, our backyard being the only place I felt comfortable swimming due to my ever-increasing weight. Taking a break from the contemporary fiction I'd been focused on reading for more than a decade, I decided to shift the focus of my reading to poetry. I was sitting there in the pool, a book of poems dangling over the edge above the comparatively dry grass, wondering why I had avoided poetry for so long (I had read it as a matter of course in undergrad; I'd even been required to write some in a first-year creative writing workshop, but since that time I had given poetry a wide berth).

Overhearing Jennifer and Nathanael playing in the yard somewhere behind me, I turned to see Jennifer set a plastic ball on top of the rubber baseball tee Nathanael had just received for his birthday. I watched in stunned silence as she stepped up to the tee and swung the oversized plastic bat. The ball rocketed into the raspberries, much to Nathanael's delight. Jennifer turned to me and smiled, proud of her line drive. I felt like I was going to faint and slip beneath the surface of the pool. "You bat *left*?!"

"Do I?" she laughed, shrugging.

Nathanael retrieved the ball from the raspberries, and Jennifer set the ball on the tee again. Instructing her to clear her head and just do what felt natural, I made her address the ball again. It was shocking to me that you could be in a committed relationship with someone for over ten years — four of those years married and cohabiting — and not be aware that they batted left.

And suddenly I was rising from the water, forsaking a towel, heedless of who might be peeking from neighbouring homes to see my stretch-marked gut and distended torso. I lumbered across the yard and up the back steps, leaving a trail of wet footprints all the way upstairs and down the hall to my office, and I banged out a poem — a poem that had come to me as a single, unified thought, as if breathed into me, a gift. The poem is called "A History of Baseball" and it was published a few days later by an online journal *Poetry Super Highway* — after years of rejections with fiction, it was the first work of any kind that had been accepted.

Acceptance had an obvious effect. I was revisiting poets I had read and enjoyed in anthologies in my undergraduate years — John Berryman, James Dickey, John Ashbery, and Michael Ondaatje — and discovering poets like Franz Wright, James Tate, Lucia Perillo, and Ken Babstock. At the same time, I was writing and submitting poems at a feverish rate and racking up a fair number of acceptances.

In 2009, just five years after writing "The History of Baseball," my first collection of poetry, *Something Burned Along the Southern Border*, was published by Mansfield Press. Jennifer and I cried at the dinner table when I took the call from editor Stuart Ross, telling me the collection would be published. Our tears scared the children, who at six, three, and two, could not yet tell tears of grief from tears of joy. We cried for the achievement. But we also cried because my mom, two years gone by that time, had not lived to see it happen. That book was shortlisted for the Gerald Lampert Memorial Award for the best first collection of poetry by a Canadian poet. It was followed by a second collection, also published by Mansfield, *Campfire Radio Rhapsody*, in 2011.

Although I find much to be proud of in both collections, I know that at their core, they are really just two books spun out of the same creative period, and I struggled going forward as a poet, trying to figure out where my poetry should go from here. There were poet friends who thought my work needed to take on a more rigorous academic tone, tackle a specific social ill or cultural shortcoming head on. And there were other poet friends who believed a more organic, laid-back approach was best: "The next book is the next book."

I appreciated the relaxed and open-minded set of this second approach but was conscious of the eyes of certain poetry gatekeepers who wanted to see the big leap forward in form and substance and poetic maturity. I found the push and pull totally paralyzing as a writer. There are poems in my two published collections about my mother's illness and death, and poems about the surreal moments of being a print journalist at a small county newspaper; there are absurdist poems born out of workshop exercises that worked out particularly well and poems about being a father, a film lover, a sober alcoholic. Looking at all the different works, I really wasn't sure what my poetry was about, and it would be years before I recognized a certain yearning, spiritual subtext in many of the poems and came to a deeper understanding of my own poetry.

But in the meantime, I was just happy to be published.

o   o   o

Early in my sobriety, a person who had been sober longer than I had been alive told me to write down where I wanted to be in five years and where I wanted to be in ten years — personally, financially, creatively, whatever. I'd written down that in five years I wanted to have a published book and more healthy children and a happy marriage. In ten years, I wrote that I wanted to have a second published book. I had no illusions about the income-earning potential of writing poetry, but at the time, however meagre the income it provided was, poetry was the breadwinner of my literary output, and I was happy with the humble gains it provided. In the first eight years of my sobriety, I had accomplished all that I thought possible in ten. Just being a present husband and father to three beautiful children — just being alive and well enough to have a life — was more than enough.

I had achieved, or so I thought, some kind of self-satisfaction, an ideal sobriety.

Years passed — good years, full of family, decent work as a journalist, and regular contact with other alcoholics. I was recovering. Every aspect of my life improved, but I could not get my eating and weight under control.

I told people being sober made me comfortable in my own skin, but my skin kept expanding to meet an ever widening and more delusional definition of comfort.

It had never been a mystery to me what I needed to do in order to lose weight. People always assume that people with weight and eating problems don't know, for example, that bread is full of sugar; that eating late at night is not a good eating habit; that eating four cheeseburgers in the car on the way home from work, throwing the wrappers in a garbage can in an alley two blocks from the house, walking in the door and eating two huge helpings of supper, then killing off the leftovers while watching sports highlights at midnight is wildly unhealthy.

I grew up with a mother who was a registered nurse and who, at one point, also worked in a health food store/restaurant. My parents were healthy, active people. I was taught how to cook and get around in a kitchen at a very young age. Things like cookies, chips, pop, and sugary cereals were not allowed in our home. It was only during our annual trip to a cottage up north that my parents would allow us to partake. The irony is, through their efforts to ensure we had a healthy diet, they were, unwittingly, creating a monster.

As I got older and started visiting friends' homes, I was shocked to learn that other families had whole cupboards dedicated to cookies, chips, and snack foods — these pantries my friends reacted to with indifference. Exposure to what was, at my house, forbidden fruit had made them immune to its delicious charms — charms I was helpless to resist.

I knew how calories worked, of course, and I knew that the physiological formula of weight loss is actually pitifully simple: burn more energy than you consume. The hard part is not what's in the fridge or in the frying pan or on your plate. The hard part is changing your thinking and behaviour. And there is no simple formula for doing that.

Another thing people assume about people with weight and overeating issues is that all we do is eat junk food and cake and meals out of the hot-'n'-ready case at 7-Eleven. But I was just as likely to open the fridge and kill a giant salad and an entire container of baba ghanoush between breakfast and lunch. My problem was a lack of *moderation*. My willpower wanted me to *consume*. Eating made me feel normal. Overeating made me feel safe, serene, and in control. All delusions, of course. Jennifer's continued attempts to change our family's eating habits, her nurturing attempts to get everyone, including three elementary school–aged children, on board with healthy eating only caused further clandestine rebellion on my part — eating in the car and at my desk at work.

There were some very short-lived attempts to lose weight and get in shape over the years. One or two of them included very brief and much less than half-assed explorations of running. In the spring of 2010, Jennifer joined the Learn to Run Clinic — a group fitness experience that, given my self-consciousness about my physical state, seemed totally unsuitable. But somehow, through gentle persuasion and feminine wiles, Jennifer was able to convince me to join her on a couple of walk/run laps of Willistead Park.

"I thought this could be something we could do together," she said, pitching me on the idea one night after the kids were in bed. "I know that you are unhappy, and I want to be healthier, too, so I thought if you ran with me, we could work on this together and help each other."

Not yet at my heaviest, but certainly well above three hundred pounds, I agreed to join her. But standing on the sidewalk in front of the house, I was in tears, paralyzed by fear because I knew, having peeked at the walk/run program schedule, that there were going to be periods of running — two-minute intervals at the most — ahead of us.

"You're not going to die," Jennifer said, full of the gentle reassurance that, in movies, always seems to presage calamity.

"You don't know that," I managed, through genuine tears.

"You're being ridiculous," she said. "You don't need to bring your phone."

Despite her protestations, I insisted on bringing it, so she could call an ambulance when I died. Obviously, neither of us died.

And I did run, without regularity or enthusiasm, for a couple of months. But I never curbed my eating, never lost any appreciable amount of weight, and, not surprisingly, never went beyond the very early reaches of the walk/run program. (It was during these early and abortive forays into running I first learned that an important lesson about weight loss: exercise isn't enough; you have to change how you eat — you can't continue to consume enough food for three or four people in the course of a day.)

This half-assed walk/run experiment came to an end while cottaging on the Bruce Peninsula. A slight roll of the ankle on a rutted road resulted in some minor tenderness and provided all the excuse I needed to proclaim that running was dangerous.

A few days after the incident with my ankle, we decided on a family hike to the Grotto — a rocky cliff overlooking a marine cave on the Georgian Bay side of the Bruce Peninsula, accessible only by a winding, wilderness trail. I wasn't in any shape for the 1.5-kilometre hike and quickly fell behind Jennifer and the kids. I was sweaty and exhausted, struggling to move over the uneven terrain. My feet were sliding around in the beach sandals I'd worn. My sore ankle began to throb. I was being passed by groups of tourists with their pricey cameras, young mothers holding babies to their breast, elderly couples walking arm in arm. Eventually, I just sat on a boulder and waited, bloated with self-loathing and self-pity.

Jennifer and the kids made it to the Grotto, but after I failed to materialize, they turned back and found me on the rock. Jennifer took one look at me, overheated and pitiful, and moved on with the kids in tow. I got up to follow, but in the twenty minutes or so I had been sitting on the boulder, my foot and ankle had swelled up, noticeably, in my sandal. I took the sandals off and tried to traverse the trail barefoot, but my pace was slowed by sharp sticks, stones, and my defeatist attitude. I felt like curling up trailside and just waiting for the rescue chopper or a team of junior rangers with a litter or the inevitable end, waiting and waving people past — *Just leave me; I am too heavy.*

Nathanael came back for me. I saw him making his determined way against the flow of traffic on the trail. He was all of eight, and the sight of his father, winded, wounded, and near tears moved him. He was too small to support me, but he tried. Just having him nearby helped me make it back to the parking lot. I heaved myself into the van, grateful that Nathanael had come back to get me and fuming that I had been led down the path then left there. The best thing for my injured ankle and pride, I knew, was rest and food.

Where the earlier mishap while running on the rutted road had done only minor damage to my ankle, the Grotto Incident, as it came to be known, had resulted in more significant tissue damage, and this "injury" lingered, becoming an additional reason — from where I stood, at least — for not losing weight and improving my health for over two years. (I kept buried the fear that I was too out of shape to get into shape.) I can't help but think my less than half-hearted effort torpedoed Jennifer's interest in running, which had been fuelled, in part by her interest in getting me active and pushing me back from the precipice my obesity had pushed me to. Soon after she completed the nine-week Learn to Run Clinic, likely sick of my litany of excuses, she stopped running, too.

o o o

The stress test booked for January 3, 2013, was not going to be my first. I'd been sent for one five and a half years earlier, in July 2007, after passing out in a friend's car. At the time, I was headed across the border with my friend Matt to eat some ridiculously spicy food at Pi's Thai in Hazel Park, Michigan.

Matt popped a bootleg copy of a Dane Cook stand-up routine into his CD player. (Please note, this was a year or so before Dane Cook was ubiquitous.) We were sitting in traffic waiting to turn into the entrance to the toll lanes for the Windsor-Detroit tunnel when Cook made a joke about the material they pave parking garages with — "How you can be going five miles per hour *in reverse* and it still sounds like a chase scene from the classic television cop show *CHiPS*?" He emulated the throaty, shrieking sound of rubber tires on parking garage floors.

It was surprisingly funny and caught me off guard. I remember bending forward in the passenger seat, laughing. And then as I sat back, still laughing, eyes closed, I experienced a full body buzz and felt like I was floating away. My eyes opened. My head was back against the headrest. The audience was laughing. Dane Cook was talking about something else.

I put my hand on Matt's arm and said, "Did something just happen there?"

We were still held up in traffic; he was busy watching for an opportunity to turn into the tunnel plaza. But when he turned and looked at me, I saw him grow concerned. He could tell I was scared. I hit the back button on the CD player, and found Dane Cook shrieking like a car in a parking garage. We let the CD play out. It took forty-two seconds for Dane Cook to say anything I recognized.

I looked at Matt: "I think I passed out for forty-two seconds."

"Passed out?" He was incredulous. "From what?!"

The obvious answer, which neither of us wanted to acknowledge, was *from Dane Cook.*

The rest of our trip across the border passed under a cloud of deep worry and paranoia. We ate at Pi's Thai in nervous silence. I dialed back the heat in my food considerably and didn't enjoy it. We laugh about it now and refer to it as the Conjoined Panic Attack, but at the time, I wasn't aware of the effect my worries, my fear, and my negativity about my weight and my health was having on others; it was overpowering the nurturing and caring nature of friends and causing them to suffer as well.

Two days later, I was once again standing, terrified, in Dr. Sijan's office. "I passed out in my friend's car from laughing," I told him.

He knew who he was dealing with, even in sobriety. "Your problem, Robert," he said "is that you are a writer. You writers, you artists, are all the same — you think too much. You spend too much time up here," he said, tapping his temple "and not enough time out here." He gestured around his examination room but was presumably referring to the world at large. "The other problem is, you weigh over three hundred pounds."

He listened to my heart and lungs, looked into my eyes and ears, checked my reflexes, palpated my abdomen and the glands in my neck. He stepped back and smiled wanly. "Robert, I think this was nothing more than a laughter-induced syncope. You fainted. You laughed very hard, very suddenly, your heart needed to make a quick correction, so it knocked you out. It is not common, but it is not harmful. I think you are okay. I would like to send you for a stress test anyway. All of this, Robert — all of these worries and the stress on your heart and your Type 2 diabetes — all of this would go away if you lost the weight."

He handed me a referral for a stress test. As he was leaving the examination room, he paused at the door, turned back, and asked, "Robert, what did you say the name of that comedian was again?"

"Dane Cook," I told him.

He wrote it down on his script pad, nodded curtly, and disappeared down the hall. Several months later, I was back in Dr. Sijan's office for some other complaint, not a single ounce lighter, and he said "Hey, that Dane Cook guy really took off, eh?"

A few days after that, I had my first stress test. The cardiologist looked at my results, gleaned from a few, hot minutes of walking on the treadmill, and told me I had fallen well short of the maximum stress level for someone my age (even for someone of my weight, which, at the time, was probably around 330 pounds). He said he could tell by the way my heart recovered from the "workout" that there was essentially nothing wrong with me outside of my abysmal physical condition.

I accepted what he told me, but I made no attempt to change my trajectory. I knew I wasn't done with food.

o   o   o

Five years later, in August 2012, Jennifer and I travelled with the children to a cottage on Oxbow Lake in the Muskokas. Sobriety had been good to me. Clearly too good. This is likely when I was at my heaviest. Our poor bathroom scale wasn't even capable of weighing me accurately at the time, though it's very likely I weighed over 370 pounds. I was far from happy.

Puffed up on some middling success with my writing, comfortable to the point of torpor in my newspaper career, loved and therefore secure at home, I was able to delude myself into believing I was comfortable in my own skin. *A gift of sobriety!* I would say. I really should have been proclaiming: *I am totally unwilling to change this one glaringly obvious thing about myself!* This, I knew, was not a quality sobriety. I knew — because I could not stand the thought or sight of myself, nor the thought of how I must appear to others, nor could I sit comfortably on most furniture, or find clothes that didn't chafe against my sweaty corpulence — that I was far from being comfortable with my physical form.

Their minds ignited by cartoons, comics, mystery novels, and films about wizards, intergalactic heroes, and time-travelling cowboys, Nathanael and Jonah (ten and seven years old at the time) had been pressing for a canoe adventure since our arrival at Oxbow Lake. I'd been putting them off, citing various reasons: I was tired, I was reading, I was writing, I wasn't sure if there were enough life jackets.

The real reason, of course, was that I was so overweight and out of shape that I was terrified of getting out into the lake and being unable to paddle back, or worse, keeling over dead in the canoe in front of my horrified sons while my wife and daughter watched helpless from the dock. Or, worse still, reaching some interesting site or brief portage along the lake's perimeter and expiring in a heap in the woods, leaving the boys, again bereft and terrified, to fend for themselves in black bear country.

But our time at Oxbow Lake was winding down. I didn't want to be a bad father, distant and inactive (the kind of father I hypocritically sat in judgment of). I, myself, had been raised by a father who had *always* been game for canoe trips and hikes and boat rides. So, despite my better judgment and fears about safety and my fitness-level, we set out in the canoe on our last full day at the cottage.

Our destination was located at the southern end of the western arm of horseshoe-shaped Oxbow Lake: a rock-strewn glade in the woods, crisscrossed with streams of water that trickled through the trees, bound for the open lake, having passed beneath a road-topped culvert from Little Oxbow Lake above. The plan was to haul the canoe ashore when we arrived at the lakehead, explore the watery glade with its fallen trees and hillocks of spongy land, thick with lichen, moss, and pine needles, and then head back.

Nathanael and Jonah took to calling us the Krapp Brothers — they considered it a scandalous pun, only allowable in the loose atmosphere of cottage time — based on the names of a pair of children's entertainers/wildlife adventurers they had watched on television when they were younger.

When we reached the embankment that led up through thick brush to West Oxbow Lake Road, the boys asked if we could continue on. Crossing the road, they said, would be like something the hero would do in a spy film or war movie; we would be forced to move with extreme caution and maximum sneakiness to avoid detection from whoever our enemy was. On that particular day, heat, the rough terrain, and my laboured breathing were our enemy.

We were never more than a kilometre away from the cottage, but it was as if we'd travelled a great distance and had fallen off the grid. The boys were having a blast; their imaginations were shooting off sparks of wacky and improbable scenarios that I knew I should have been enjoying. But I was sweaty, sore, and feeling a familiar sensation of panic starting up in my chest and head. *Were my lips buzzy? Was I lightheaded? Was my left arm numb?* We'd better head back.

And head back we did. Without incident, even. And it was as we paddled into view of where Jennifer and Thomasin waited for us on the dock that Jennifer snapped a photo with her smartphone of Nathanael, Jonah, and me paddling back from our adventure. In the photo, the canoe rides dangerously low. I'm seated in the middle. Not on the yoke but down in the hull. To have me seated at the stern with a sixty-pound Jonah or even a one-hundred-pound Nathanael up front would have seen the bow raised several feet out of the water; the reverse seating arrangement was not feasible if travel was the goal. So, the boys paddled, Nathanael steering with some difficulty, while I rode along shouting out directions. A cask of humanity in a comically small life jacket, I would surely have dragged to the bottom like a pocket square had we capsized. (I swam freestyle and breaststroke in Southwestern Ontario regional championships in high school. Would I have been able to swim one hundred metres to the dock?) In the photo, I have a paddle, and even though the water is lapping at the gunwales, under the strictures of the life jacket, I could not reach across my own girth to even lily-dip the tip of the blade.

The photo, of course, shows all of this in one horrifying, frozen moment.

"Awww, look at my boys, back from their adventure," Jennifer sang once we had beached ourselves and I had tumbled from the canoe on near-cataleptic legs and made it safely to the dock.

I took one look at the photo on the screen of Jennifer's phone, and it ruined whatever part of my day hadn't already been sullied by not being able to give Nathanael and Jonah a full Krapp Brothers adventure because of my immobility and fear. I asked her to delete it.

"Oh, but the boys look so happy," she said, enlarging their faces on her screen. "Look at those smiles! Oh, my heart is melted."

I scrolled the photo over to me. I looked utterly helpless and incapacitated sitting in that canoe. I looked old. I looked like a clown. I looked enormous. Here I had been wasting so much mental energy worried about scarring my children with an ugly death when what I should have been worried about was embarrassing them because I was alive. I was crushed. And although that photo played a role in the endgame of my eating and obesity, it was not the end — not yet.

○   ○   ○

That fall, the Afghan Whigs played a reunion tour show at Saint Andrew's Hall in Detroit. The Whigs, and, in particular, their seminal 1993 album, *Gentlemen*, had played an important role in our early courting, and Jennifer and I were excited about seeing these debonair sons of Cincinnati for the first time in nearly twenty years. We arranged for a babysitter and headed across the border to the show. We saw a ton of people we knew; the Whigs were tremendous, and then came the ride home.

Jennifer and I were walking across Congress Street in Detroit, heading to where we parked, when I had to reach out for her arm to steady myself.

"Holy shit, my feet," I said, lurching to the curb and holding onto a signpost. "They're killing me."

"They're probably just asleep from standing for so long," Jennifer said, trying to coax me along so we could get home and relieve Molly, the babysitter. She was probably partially right. We had been on our feet for more than three hours, moving very little on the hot, crowded ballroom floor. In the short distance we'd travelled out onto the street, circulation had returned to my lower extremities, but with that came extreme cramping. It felt like my feet were trying to fold themselves in half inside of my shoes. By the time we'd covered the expanse of the parking lot, I could barely walk; each step was agony, and my breathing was ragged and laboured. I was behind the wheel when we drove into the Windsor-Detroit Tunnel and hit a traffic slowdown.

Thrombosis. The unspoken fear of every working journalist, whether they are two hundred pounds overweight, or not. The long hours spent seated before multiple screens, monitoring news feeds, cranking out and editing copy, laying out pages; the failure to stand up and allow blood to circulate freely and naturally through your legs — they provided an open invitation to it. And then, there it was: a monstrous clot of blood building up in the vasculature behind your knee, waiting for the express lane to your heart; sudden, unbearable pain, vermillion eruption from the mouth, the lifeless collapse … It had found me. At an Afghan Whigs concert in Detroit, of all places, but thrombosis cares not for your musical taste. It just wants to cripple you with hurt before it drops you.

"We need to switch places," I pleaded with Jen. "You take off your seatbelt and climb over top to here, and I will take off my seatbelt and slide under to your side."

"We're moving!"

"Yeah, but we're not going that fast!" I was crying out with each acceleration and sudden braking as they required the use of my feet as traffic crawled south into Canada. "I shouldn't be driving. What if something happens? C'mon, we can do this!"

We didn't do it. I composed myself enough to make it through Canada Customs without having to give the Customs official too long-winded an explanation as to why my brow was bathed in sweat and furrowed in anguish and just what these "Afghanistani Wigs," as he called them, gesturing about his head, were. When we pulled up in front of the house it was just before midnight. I had some special instructions for Jennifer:

"Go inside and make sure the kids are sleeping and send Molly home," I gasped. "Then I will get into the house."

"I can help you into the house," Jennifer said. It was clear she thought I was being very dramatic and silly.

"Just go," I said hoarsely, not wanting my wife to witness what, given my pain levels, could possibly be my final throes, my shoes kicking around spasmodically in the foot well. I heaved my legs around and, sitting on the edge of the driver's seat, attempted to loosen my shoes laces. Bending over that far was usually a chore any-way; at that point, I was struggling more than ever and my breathing was ragged. I dropped to my knees in the road beside the van and crawled into the gutter. Jen was just mounting the front porch.

"Tell her I haven't been drinking!" I called out. "Tell her some-thing is wrong with my feet!"

Jennifer disappeared into the house, and I began crawling, frantically, across the lawn toward the front porch. I could just imagine the neighbours, including Molly's mother across the street, watching me from behind the edge of a curtain, believing they were witnessing first-hand what the end of nearly a decade of sobriety looks like.

I made it to the porch and took a seat on the cold cement steps, acting as if I was enjoying the brisk evening air as Molly skipped out the door, down the steps, and across the street like a gazelle.

"She didn't see me, did she?" I asked. "Crawling across the lawn?" I indicated the muddied, grass-stained knees of my jeans.

"Why are you worried Molly would think you were drinking?" Jennifer asked.

"Well, I'm assuming the last time I was so drunk I had to crawl in the door she was probably five or six years old and long asleep in bed, so I don't want this to be her lasting memory of the last time she ever babysat for us because of the condition I came home in."

Jennifer laughed and held the door open as I crawled into the house.

Now the moment of horrific truth: "I need you to help get my shoes off," I said, in a grave whisper, not wanting to alert the children to my plight — they were supposed to be sleeping, but we could hear them scurrying around and giggling upstairs, excited to hear about the concert but also pretending to be asleep. My feet throbbed in their leather sarcophagi. I didn't know what to expect: swollen vessels, corpuscular and purple, ready to burst and spill toxins, as if bitten by adders; or mangled, atrophied husks, all but snapping off when my shoes were removed. I couldn't bear to watch.

There was some sweet agony of relief as Jennifer pulled off my shoes and socks. "How are they?" I asked, laying back on the stairs, an arm draped across my eyes.

"They are fine," Jennifer said. "They stink," she said, trying to lighten the mood, "but they look normal."

I pleaded with her not to make me laugh as the jiggling of my flesh dialed up the pain in my feet. I looked down to where Jennifer held my one foot in her hands. Other than the hard indentation of where my sock had been pressing into my ankle, they looked normal. Deceptively normal, I decided.

Though the pain subsided, I spent a largely sleepless night waiting for the blood clot to kill me where I lay.

◦ ◦ ◦

A month later, I was waking up from that sweat-soaked nap that followed my two laps of Willistead Park. I paced around the kitchen, enumerating all the ways I was going to change and all the reasons I had for doing it. I told Jennifer about the miscommunication with Dr. Hanson and how, before my appointment on January 3, I was going to lose weight and get in shape so that when I had the stress test, I would ace it. None of this "Okay, you didn't die, but you didn't really pass, either" kind of bullshit I had been satisfied with after my laughter-induced syncope.

"You know, my mom wanted me to promise her when she was lying in the hospital that I would lose weight," I said to Jennifer, choking up. "She knew she was dying. I knew she was dying — I'm not sure anybody else knew, but I knew she was dying. Five months later, she was dead, and I hadn't done anything about it. I couldn't even promise her I would try. Do you know what I said to her? Do you know what I said sitting there, to my dying mother, when all she wanted for me was that I lose weight and get healthy? I said, 'I don't have time.' That's the kind of son I was. That's the kind of son I am. And I don't want to be that way anymore."

Jennifer was now crying, and she hugged me, and we stood there in the living room. "You are not that to me," she said. "And your mom loved you so much. But you do have the time if you want to have it. I will help."

My goal, I stated that night, sitting on the stairs, staring Jen right in the eye, was to lose one hundred pounds by my fortieth birthday. I had nineteen months to go.

CHAPTER FOUR

THE BIG THAW

THERE'S A REASON why those mismatched active wear coordinates — the ones that made me look like an extra in a second-rate film about third-rate mafia hangers-on — had been languishing in my dresser drawers all those long, lonely years. They were about to get the shit worked out of them.

I started walking every day. It was the onset of winter, and whether I got up early in the morning, or went out late at night, I walked every day for thirty-seven straight days. The walks got longer and longer. With the exception of the two years I spent in Montreal as a student, I had lived in Windsor — in the same neighbourhood — my entire life. To my surprise, I discovered there were places in Windsor that I just didn't know existed. My walks took me into parts of the city I had never seen before: heretofore unknown residential cul-de-sacs; derelict light industry nooks and hidden commercial crannies; whole tracts of new homes where, previously, I hadn't even imagined fields. Waylaid and blindfolded and dropped off in some of these locales, I would have assumed I was in some other town. But on foot, I saw better how the unfamiliar streets and hidden neighbourhoods connected to the city I knew all too well.

I came to realize that beyond the actual physical movement, a big part of why walking was working for me — and the reason why countless gym memberships failed in the past — is that I need *visual stimulation*. There are walkers and runners for whom walking and running means heading down to the treadmill placed in front of a large-screen television in their basements; there are others for whom it means circling the rubber-surfaced tracks at their gym. I've tried treadmills out of curiosity, and once, during a snowstorm, I went to Jennifer's gym as a guest to try the indoor track. I found both completely beyond the pale of boredom. If confronted with a fitness regimen that out of some nightmarish necessity required me to run entirely on a treadmill or indoor track, I would be buried in a piano crate, also out of necessity. Walking and running in place, or on an oval track are, to me, tantamount to stasis. By the time desperation got me walking, I was fucking done with stasis. In order for me to evolve and change the trajectory of my life, I actually had to changing my location with each step.

The long, exploratory walks that served as the prerequisite to my running career provided some insight into this theory of visual stimulus. It wasn't only *my* movement that mattered; there had to be a corresponding movement of the landscape, architecture, and traffic moving past and around me. Seeing the city where I had lived nearly my entire life from different directions and below the speed of traffic; knowing that the driveway on Kildare Road across the street from my parents' friends Bob and Mary Lou Taylor's house was exactly 2.5 kilometres from my front door; seeing a collection of shopfronts that I had never seen before; recognizing, from one outing to the next, the same clutch of fishermen in the same spot along the railing along the riverfront trails … I was taking it all in; my imagination was engaged.

The newly revealed strangeness of the city, and of walking in general, kept me interested. I wandered farther and farther, discovering strange and new places, but I always found my way home. At the time, I had no way to measure the distances I was walking, so, once home, I would jump in the van, set the trip odometer, and drive back over the route, marking the date and distance walked on a calendar hanging in my home office.

○ ○ ○

The weight began to come off. But it wasn't just because of the walking (and driving around in a Dodge Caravan measuring distances with the odometer). Eating was how I got myself into this mess, and eating was definitely going to have to be part of the solution. I was going to have to disabuse myself of the thought that food and overeating were offering me any real comfort. I had been on many diets and weight-loss programs over the years, but any success I had while on them was barely worth discussing, as it was quickly overtaken and defiled by my insatiable appetites.

In denying myself that final gorging at Motorburger, in opting instead to take a walk around Willistead Park, I had surrendered that one stubborn shred of my willpower to that same Higher Power who delivered me from my alcoholism. I had finally come to a reckoning with my diseased relationship with food and eating that in its destructiveness resembled in many ways my relationship with alcohol.

Despite the similarities, there was one striking difference between my abuse of alcohol and my overeating: where my drinking was always a very public, ego-driven, shameless affair, a lot of my worst eating took place in secret — hidden from my family, co-workers, and friends, I gorged on extra meals and an endless array of snacks, all served with a side of self-opprobrium.

Drinking, strangely, is more socially acceptable than overeating. In my case, I think this was largely due to the fact that when I was drinking, I was usually with people who for the most part drank the way I drank, and the atmosphere when we drank was elevated and convivial. It was a party. Drunkenness was not only expected; it was *the point*.

Eating also happened in these situations, of course, but because it was a party, all the usual restrictions and expectations were loosened, just as with alcohol. But obviously most of my eating for sustenance didn't take place around the same people I drank with. It took place at home, or in professional settings where there are expected levels of moderation, etiquette, etc., levels of moderation that I regularly failed to meet — often in spectacular fashion. This failure was something I was acutely aware of, as it came to form the basis for people's expectations of how I was going to behave around food, i.e., that I would make a pig of myself. This was particularly problematic when I was sober and still eating like crazy. And even though I was horribly self-conscious about people seeing me overeating, the pain caused by that was nowhere near intolerable enough to put my gluttony in check. As a result, there were, sadly, many witnesses of my out-of-control feasting. And those who didn't see my eating with their own eyes would have heard stories — in fact, I know there were stories: I circulated many of them myself, out of some grim need to get out ahead of the narrative by fulfilling the role of the self-deprecating obese man. Whether or not people saw me or heard of my gluttony, it was hard to hide that fact that there was a problem since the results of my overeating were always there in my weight gain.

I had experience quitting drinking and getting sober; changing my relationship with food was difficult in different and unexpected ways. Whereas achieving sobriety requires 100 percent abstinence from alcohol and drugs, you *have to* eat to survive. And Western custom dictates that you eat three times a day at prescribed times.

A sober friend who also struggles with food and eating issues put it this way: "When you are sober, your alcoholism becomes like a tiger you have locked in a cage for which you have thrown away the key. You never plan on opening that door. When you are spiritually fit, the tiger is docile, kitten-like, sleeping softly in a corner of the cage. When you are agitated and living on willpower, the tiger is agitated, scratching at the bars, bloodthirsty ... But as long as you don't open the cage door, you are safe. The tiger cannot harm you, and once you do all the things you need to do to maintain your sobriety, the tiger returns to that serene state.

"With eating and food, you put the tiger in the cage, but at least three times a day you have to take the tiger out of the cage, feed it, and then successfully put it back in the cage, all without getting smitten by its disarming cuteness or mauled because it tricked you with its disarming cuteness."

So, what I did was start to eat very *deliberately*. I looked at every meal as a distinct event. I ate with mindfulness and awareness, sitting at a table with my meal in front of me wherever possible, thinking about what I was doing: chewing, swallowing, allowing myself to feel full but also *satisfied* (an eating experience I was sadly unfamiliar with). Not every meal was a communal event, but I wasn't sneaking away from my desk at the newspaper to sit alone in my van in a parking lot eating enough lunch for everyone in the newsroom. I prepared lunches at home in advance. I limited snacks to fruits, modest portions of crackers and cheese, and healthy handfuls of nuts. My days of killing containers of leftovers and handfuls of cake over the sink were over.

My Scottish roots had bred into me a love of oatmeal, and I upped my morning intake of oatmeal and other high-fibre cereals, while reducing the carbs and refined sugars I usually ingested in the mornings in the form of cold cereals and toast. I also cut out the selection of pastries I usually ordered with my morning coffee takeout. In fact, any breads I ate were multi-grain or high-fibre Bavarian ryes. I became a regular at Windsor's two premium salad bars, avoided high-sodium foods like soup, and increased my intake of lean, unprocessed proteins, like poultry or fish. Amongst my friends, I became something of a laughingstock for my go-to snacks of what are sometimes called "poop fruit": figs, prunes, and dates.

Considering the kitchen "closed" after supper was a healthy-eating practice my mother had tried to instill in me. Inadvertently, though, she created a child who snuck food out of the kitchen cupboards late at night and ate the food in the darkest corners of the basement. A crucial step in altering my eating habits and curbing my weight gain was to stop eating after supper. Leftovers began surviving long enough to fulfill their intended purpose: eaten the next day for lunch, or even as supper two nights in a row, rather than dying a quick, late-night death over the kitchen sink while sports highlights droned on in the background.

Food also stopped being my go-to reward for things I fancied myself having achieved. Apparently, I thought being a published poet working at a county weekly was worthy of deep-fried laurels and garlands of cured meats at every turn because these rewards and those like them were always finding their way into my gullet. *Survived another day at my desk talking to people on the phone? That's an eight dried-pepperette achievement! Turned a fine phrase at the end of a hard-fought stanza? Have you tried these new salt & vinegar kettle chips? Yes? Well, have you tried a whole family-sized bag?*

I needed a new carrot. (And don't worry, as a father of three children, I wasn't about to use those ridiculous baby carrots that look like they have been turned on a lathe.) No, instead I turned to the reward that had been right in front of me since my first experimentations with it in tenth grade, when sleepless nights extended into sweaty, hyper-aware days: the calorie-free rabbit hole of fine coffees and espresso. I'm not sure I actually increased my caffeine intake, which is probably a small mercy, but I did start *using* coffee differently, spacing out my doses more judiciously, so they coincided with the beats of the workday or evening writing binges, when I would have typically thrown down an entire sleeve of Saltines thick with peanut butter and jam, or polished off a couple bowls of cereal to mark a completed task, I would treat myself to a fine Ethiopian Yirgacheffe or a Sumatran Mandheling coffee or a series of fast espressos at my favourite cafe along Erie Street. I kept track of everything I ate in a small notebook, assigning values learned during past dalliances with weight-loss programs to everything I ate. Eventually, I migrated everything over to a food-tracking, weight-loss app on my smartphone.

Although visits to restaurants were steeply curtailed, I did eventually return to Motorburger, going with Jennifer and the kids. The owners, old friends, prepared a special, off-menu turkey burger for me, topped with spinach on a gluten-free bun, and served with a large salad on the side.

Putting the lessons of the errored-out scale to good use, we bought a digital scale rated to four hundred pounds. I weighed myself every morning, standing naked in the bathroom. Each day's weight was recorded on a big pad of paper kept in the linen closet in our upstairs hallway. Even if I couldn't see the weight coming off in the mirror or feel it in the way my clothes fit my body, I could at least see it moving in increments on the page, and I began obsessively chasing the numbers. I would play games, pitting myself against the scale, seeing if I could guess the next day's loss, right down to the 0.2-pound (approximately three-ounce) increments reported by the digital scale. I would challenge myself to reach a certain weight by the weekend, or by the end of the month. It quickly became a preoccupation.

And just as quickly I learned that weight loss is a long game, and it's as much about patience and accepting strange upticks despite good portion control, exercise, and water intake, as it is about seeing the hard-won downticks. There were days when something like the salt content of a single, small bowl of hot and sour soup made me gain seven pounds of retained water. And days when I ate clean and lean but found the next morning that the numbers on the scale went in the wrong direction because the body's natural response to not being fed what it has been conditioned to expect is to put calories into reserve and hang on to weight.

I don't necessarily recommend these mental math games as the best way to go about losing weight, but it kept me interested in what was happening to my body. Although I was often wrong in my estimating, I approached each day with optimism — I always expected to lose weight and would look back on the previous day's activity levels, hydration, and, of course, food intake to learn what was working and what was not.

Over longer stretches of time, I was struck by how I could see and feel the results of even incremental weight loss (sometimes a matter of ounces) both physically and mentally. Yet, when I had been gaining weight steadily and detrimentally over the better part of the two preceding decades, it had been next to impossible for me to recognize the effects; I was blinded by the intoxication of willpower and the fantasy world of denial.

Soon, with daily walks — often between 8 and 10 kilometres in length — daily weigh-ins, a high-fibre, high-protein, low-carb diet, and not touching any food after supper, there was no denying I was losing weight. I was certainly not achieving that loss through any act of willpower. Just as I had abandoned the diseased thinking that kept me drinking despite countless reasons not to, I abandoned the willpower that kept me eating when it was clearly killing me. There was no struggle. The fight was over, and I had lost. And there was a great feeling of relief in knowing that. I adopted a rational response to the presence of things to eat and a calculated approach to the necessity of eating. I was getting sober from food.

When I walked into that stress echocardiogram appointment on January 3, 2013, I weighed 314 pounds — fifty-four pounds less than I had on November 28.

The walls of the test area were festooned with monitors, and the Windsor Cardiac Centre's echocardiogram team was intent on the data that was being spit out of my body. I wasn't going to let them down. Although I was scared, I was going to give them something positive to analyze.

For the stress echocardiogram, the standard complement of electrodes, sensors, and wires were attached to my arms, legs, fingers and chest. They had me lie down on an examination bed next to the treadmill. "This is going to let us see what your heart looks like at work and how it behaves while at rest," one of the lab techs explained as they performed another ultrasound.

When I was fully relaxed, my heart beating at a fairly normal seventy-something beats per minute, they hauled me to my feet and got me up on the treadmill. Immediately, I was walking briskly up an incline. I flashed back to my woefully out-of-shape treadmill test I had taken after the laughter-induced syncope. I felt fear chipping away at the edges of my resolve to make this test worth the effort. And with that acknowledgement of the effort — everything I did in the preceding weeks to get myself ready for a medical test; the effort I put in, pushing myself to walk in the cold every day; my steadfastness in avoiding the constant temptation of food — I cast my fear aside and focused on the task at hand.

There is nothing to be afraid of here. Regardless of the results, only good things will come of this.

A couple of minutes into the brisk walk, I broke into a light jog. If I cracked a chamber or tore a valve, I would be in good hands.

And there was a bed to collapse on — which is what they had me do when my heart rate got up around 145 beats per minute. With my heart pounding in my chest, the technicians immediately lay me back down on the bed — shouting instructions and encouragement to each other like stevedores lowering a cask of unknown yet potentially volatile contents — and performed another echocardiogram.

That's when the cardiologist entered, like a high priest in a lab coat. He stared at the various monitors and asked for the sensor to be set at different angles so that he could better see how my heart looked under stress. I was led to a room to await the doctor and my results.

He came in and sat down, a young man of considerable carriage himself. He flipped through printouts and made some notes. He looked me up and down, confirmed my age, and then said, "Why were you referred here?"

"I was having trouble breathing," I told him. "I was scared I was going to die."

"Well, you're not going to die," he said, smiling. "At least not any time soon. I don't see any problem here, or even a reason for referral. Your heart is big and strong, and it is in very good shape for someone of your size." He paused and flipped through some pages. "I see you've lost a considerable amount of weight since your first visit. How are you doing that?"

I told him about my change in diet and about my walking. "But I'm worried," I said, "that maybe I shouldn't push any harder because maybe I am too heavy to get in shape. I worry that if I went out for a run or a bike ride, people are going to find me passed out in a ditch somewhere, and when I come-to in the hospital, the doctors are going to say 'What the hell do you think you were doing, going for a bike ride? A man of your size? You are way too heavy to get in shape.'"

"Well, I don't recommend you run; you'll injure yourself, and then you won't be able to continue," he said. "But there is no reason why you shouldn't be able to push your heart as hard as you need to in order to get to a healthy weight."

He asked if I had any questions for him. I did: "If you can't see anything in my tests, what was causing my shortness of breath, the tightness in my chest?"

And here he confirmed what doctors and counsellors, whether professional or friends, had been telling me for years. "It's in your head," he said, tapping his temple in unconscious imitation of Dr. Sijan before him. "The breathlessness, the difficulty speaking, the tightness in the chest … we make this happen with our thinking. If you continue to lose weight, your thinking will change."

These symptoms didn't just resemble the symptoms of panic attacks. They were all physical manifestations of my body being out of step with my mind, the very core of my being signalling its desperate discomfort with the physical form I was taking, and how it was ruining my life — a life I had fought so hard to wrest back from the depths of alcoholism. Just like my heart shutting down my consciousness to reset my system when I laughed too hard at a Dane Cook's parking structure bit, this was my consciousness trying to shut down my heart, to get my attention, to rattle me into change.

o   o   o

When I went out for my walk the following night, something the cardiologist had said the previous day was still bothering me. He had warned me, specifically, against running. Injury, he said, would surely find me and ruin any chance I had of shedding the rest of this weight. Once injured, I would almost certainly require a period of rest in order to rehabilitate. This would see me gain weight — a demoralizing prospect. But so far, going against my natural inclinations had paid off handsomely.

I'd had so many new holes punched in my belt over the weeks that the local leather worker had to clip excess material off the end. My pants ballooned clownishly around my waist, ass, and legs. Once-tight shirts were starting to resemble blousy smocks. I was starting to look a bit unkempt. People were starting to wonder if I was sick, coming up to me to inquire privately after my health.

And, to be completely honest, *I was getting really fucking sick of walking.*

I came to the foot of Moy Avenue and Riverside Drive. Off to my right, at the eastern terminus of the Riverfront Trail, I could see an illuminated pillar glowing blue in the misty darkness. It sat at the foot of Lincoln Road, two blocks away. I didn't allow myself too much time to think about it. The doctor at the cardiology centre was a nice guy but fuck him and what he thought I was capable of doing. I started running. It was the first time I had run outdoors in years, probably since very lightly turning my ankle on that rutted road on the Bruce Peninsula in 2010. I was slow, I was heavy, I was a little bit scared, but when I reached the glowing blue pillar at the foot of Lincoln Road, I was still upright and only a little bit winded. I decelerated into a walk and continued on with my evening constitutional. I was coming to a better understanding of moderation.

"I ran," I told Jennifer, upon walking in the door.

Now it was her turn to be scared. I could see it in her uncertain smile. Later that night, she admitted that although at one time she had cajoled me to run with her by telling me I wasn't going to die, she was now nervous.

"You've come a long way just walking," she said. "I don't want to see you get hurt and not be able to keep losing weight. It's been nice to see you so happy."

"The doctor at the cardiology place said the same thing," I told her. "He told me not to run because if I get hurt, I'll be right back where I started. But that's the kind of fear — the fear of getting hurt or having a heart attack while trying to get in shape — that stopped me from doing anything for years! I'm so tired of being afraid! It feels so good not to be!"

Jennifer understood. She understood because she knows how stubborn, how suffused with willpower I can be, even in sobriety. Often throughout our marriage she has commented on how she envies my ability, when I make up my mind to do something, to do it all the way, without compromise. It used to be that way with drinking, and it was certainly that way when I chose to get sober. She had witnessed it with my dedication to poetry and writing. It all just depended on which way I directed my stubbornness: was I digging in with my diseased self-will and cutting myself off from happiness, health, and a more spiritual path, or was I turning that willpower over and stubbornly refusing to reengage with it, letting God's will direct me? Either way, I was blessed to be married to someone who understood. Just as she'd understood when, upon entering the house earlier that night and announcing that I ran, I had immediately grabbed my keys and headed out to the van to measure the distance from the foot of Moy to the foot of Lincoln with the odometer.

As it turns out, it was 210 metres. Not much on a global scale. Not even much on a neighbourhood scale, but it was a start, and I was emboldened — I would even go so far as to say enchanted — with my ability to run, even a short distance. Each daily walk now included a brief stint of running.

On the evening of February 10, 2013, I attended a committee meeting for some service work I was involved with related to my sobriety. I still had not missed a day of walking. I weighed 303 pounds, sixty-five pounds less than I did when I started.

The meeting was being held at a friend's house. It was less than a twenty-minute walk from home, so I went on foot, using the walk as part of my daily regimen. During the meeting, it started to rain. When the meeting was done, several people offered me lifts home, but I declined. With my committee papers rolled up and stashed in the sleeve of my jacket, I set out from my friend's front porch in a freezing, steady downpour, not at a walk, but at a run.

Soaked and shivering, I stumbled in the front door of home. The rain camouflaged the fact that I was crying. Apparently, I couldn't outrun the rain, but I'd made it home, and it was overwhelming.

"I ran all the way," I wheezed. "All the way from Jim's."

Jennifer and the kids were at first concerned, but when they realized I was elated and not injured or afraid, they helped me out of my wet clothes, and bundled me up in blankets on the couch, all three kids lying down on top of me to transfer their warmth.

"I didn't even stop," I crowed, like a child convinced he's run faster and farther in new running shoes. "I've never run that far in my life!"

It was true. I had probably never run that far in a single stretch in my life. But I had no idea how far that was. I was going to need that number for the notes I was keeping — notes that would eventually become the basis of this book — so as soon as I was sufficiently warmed up, I put on fresh clothes and jumped in the van to measure the distance: 2.1 kilometres. I was floored. It didn't even seem possible. I felt like I had discovered, at thirty-eight, that I had long had the ability to fly residing, untapped, within me. The idea that I had run that far, non-stop, was just that surreal and beguiling.

◦ ◦ ◦

Running remained a cool trick that I had discovered I could do and wanted to master. The thrill of jumping in the van after each run to retrace my steps and measure the distance did, however, eventually wear off.

It took me a few days of digging, but I eventually unearthed in a dresser drawer the old Timex Ironman watch I'd had since high school — chunky digital sports watches were all the rage then, and even people who engaged in no form of physical activity wore them. I started using the watch's built-in stopwatch feature to time my runs on the courses I mapped out for myself using various online mapping apps.

I knew through reading a few running magazines that one of the base-level achievements for runners was running a 5K. It was a daunting prospect, so daunting, that in my mania for recording and chasing my stats, I couldn't leave it unchallenged. I registered at the local running store, the Running Factory, for its annual Spring Thaw 5K, printed up a beginner's 5K training schedule I found online, and started training.

The training schedule took into account things like age, weight, running experience, and goal finishing time. The plan called for eight training runs (five 3-kilometre runs and three 4-kilometre runs) over the three-week period leading up to race day. I charted out various 3- and 4-kilometre routes through the neighbourhood, giving each one a name based on the shape they made on the map, clever names like "T-Route," or the street they were predominately run on, like "Kildare Corridor."

I pasted the running schedule into the first page of my first-ever running journal, and when I returned from each run, I would take the time from my Timex Ironman, divide it by the kilometres of the pre-established route, and figure out my pace. Right away, I was gratified to see that my actual pace — initially around ten minutes per kilometre, falling to 8:23 per kilometre by the eighth training run — was quicker than the training plan's projected pace. It meant I had lowballed myself when filling out the online training plan generator's questionnaire, but I was learning to be more prudent in every aspect of my life. Overreaching, over-thinking, and over-indulging had nearly everything to do with the hedonistic mess I was trying to undo. The glacier of paralyzing self-will and fear within that was keeping me from being a better husband, father, brother, son, friend, and employee, was slowly beginning to melt.

I was learning to be a realist.

◦ ◦ ◦

It was 6:00 a.m. on March 24, 2013, and I was pacing around the living room in the semi-darkness, fuelling up with a toasted bagel with peanut butter, a banana, and honey (a combo that would become a staple of my pre-race diet). With the starting horn for the Spring Thaw still four hours away, I even went for a walk around the neighbourhood to "stay loose."

It's endearing now, my earnestness and my naïveté regarding the preparation required for a 5K, but it was my first race, and it was what I needed to do to stay calm. I didn't want to be one of those people who fake an injury or illness before an important event. I had worked hard just to be able to show up for this. I may have looked awkward and hopelessly unstylish in my motley running ensemble, but I had made a fool out of myself in public before — as a drunk thinking he was cool. Now, I cared considerably less whether or not anyone thought I was cool and considerably more about being an all-round healthier person. Accepting challenges and limitations was part of this — both things I had learned in sobriety. Running 5 kilometres in a pack of people — in broad day-light! — was going to be a challenge, but it certainly was not going to be my limit. Running was beginning to change me.

The Spring Thaw attracts about five hundred runners every year. The parking lot outside the Running Factory was set up with

registration and vendor tents; tables offered coffee, juice, doughnuts, and bagels, mostly to keep all those not running entertained
and warm once the race was underway. It was a frigid, blustery day.
Jennifer and the kids waited in the van while I did another warmup
walk around a few blocks of Olde Riverside.

A few minutes before the gun, the race announcer called for all
the participants to queue up around the corner on Villaire Street,
one block east of the Running Factory. I stood there in the throng,
uncertain of how to deal with all the nervous energy around me.
Did it augur well that everyone seemed to be as keyed up as I was,
or was it a bad omen — were we all newbs rushing headlong into
the maiming maw of the March wind?

I looked to the curb, where Jennifer and the kids stood on someone's ice-crusted front lawn, the kids eating the Timbits they'd
stuffed their pockets with at the hospitality tent. For a brief, eter-
nal second, I wanted to be there with them — colder, maybe, for
standing still, but less lonely and therefore warmer.

When the gun went off, there was a big roar from the crowd,
and people went charging north on Villaire toward Riverside Drive,
some people running up on residential lawns, hurdling hedges and
winter-blistered gardens to get ahead. At Riverside Drive, which
was blocked off to traffic for the duration of the race, the course
turned east. I was at the 2-kilometre marker — still half a kilometre
away from the turn-around pylon — when a race volunteer on a
bicycle came pedalling along ushering everyone into the eastbound
lane: "Race leaders coming through!" he bellowed. "Race leaders
coming through!"

It hardly seemed possible but seconds later a pack of runners
flashed past in silks and singlets, their skin raw in the cold. There
were many people running this race in winter coats and casual
clothes; people pushing baby strollers — this was a race to shake
out the sails, to get the lead out, to, as the race name suggested,

thaw out the legs after a long winter layoff. I had been walking and running all winter, just to make sure I could finish the race, even if I had to stumble across the finish line. But clearly, there were those who used the Spring Thaw as a 5K benchmarking exercise. These race-leading fanatics were clearly not of my lowly ilk, and possibly not of this Earth. I felt a pang of jealousy. These local elites, all full-stride and nearly naked, just made running look so effortless.

That pang was made worse by a middle-aged couple who were attacking the Spring Thaw using the walk-run method. I passed them at their leisure, very early in the race, walking hand-in-hand, in slacks, button-downs, goose-down vests, and blown-out cross trainers. Minutes later, I saw a very similarly dressed couple walking up ahead of me. When I pulled alongside, I realized it was the same couple. The man looked at his watch, barked a command, and they took off at a sprint and left me in their tracks. This was not sitting well with me. I watched as they returned to walking a few hundred metres down the road. I picked up my pace a bit and gradually closed the gap to within a few strides, but then the man's watch signalled another sprint. He barked his command, and they were off again, at a pace much faster than I was willing (or able) to hit, let alone maintain, if I wanted to finish the race.

We went back and forth like this a few times over the 5 kilometres. Turning onto Villaire Street in the final few hundred metres of the race, I spotted them up ahead of me. Jogging. They were all out of sprint, but I wasn't — and I'd be damned if I was going to let a couple in slacks who walked the majority of the race beat me. I hit speeds in that final charge down Villaire that I had not hit since I ran high-school football wind sprints. I passed them at the hardest dead sprint I could muster and made the turn onto Wyandotte Street, where people stood behind barriers, with cowbells and noise-makers, roaring encouragement at every single runner approaching the inflatable arch that marked the finish. I prayed none of the spectators would make the disastrous decision to step into the chute to visit a friend on the other side because I was not stopping — even if I had wanted to, sheer momentum was running the show now. If someone stepped in front of me, they were going to be carried across the finish line, impacted on my torso like a bug on a windshield.

Eleven weeks after taking my first uncertain strides as a runner along the Riverfront Trail, I finished my first 5K with a time of 42:50, fortieth out of forty in the 35–39-year-old male category, the 202nd male to finish overall. I was elated. Jennifer was elated. I got a medal, which impressed the hell out the kids, and along with a couple of hard-earned Timbits for the road, I grabbed a promotional flyer for the Learn to Run Clinic.

CHAPTER FIVE

THE RUNNING-SHAPED HOLE

MY ELATION AT finishing my first 5K race was short-lived. My self-satisfaction could not outpace my self-consciousness, and though I could soon see even more of my progress thanks to a phone-based running app I had been hipped to by the running magazines, I was terrified of being *seen* myself. That same fear that kept me away from the kids' school so their friends and peers, their teachers, and other parents wouldn't see what an enormous anchor on the emotional well-being of my children I had become kept me running under cover of darkness for several months.

I didn't know what I looked like running, so I had no empirical evidence that the heaving and shaking of my body was going on anywhere except in my head, but I didn't want to make it easy for anyone else to collect empirical evidence, either. The shame I felt about my physical appearance and how it was affecting my relationships with my children was enough without the eyes and judgment of the neighbourhood upon me.

Knowing first-hand how difficult it is to lose weight and being ceaselessly aware of my physical appearance despite my best efforts to be body positive, I have a special, very dark place in my personal pantheon of active resentments for anyone who body shames a runner. That special class of asshole who looks a runner up and down and judges them based on some narrow, misguided body image criteria; those withering know-it-alls who believe the only people who have any business calling themselves runners are those who conform to the exacting ectomorphic standards of the stereotypical world-class distance runner. As a bigger runner, I learned early on that I did not jibe with certain people's notions of ideal body type and height-to-weight ratio, and that, acquaintance or stranger, these people weren't going to be afraid to let me know, whether through insult, eye roll, arched eyebrow, snicker, or scoff.

Looking back, I shouldn't have been surprised, but the bureaucratic fetishism of the insurance industry only helped drive this frustrating reality home. Through my protracted, drunken adolescence, life insurance hadn't even been on my radar. But running had placed it squarely on the map before me, like a geocache prize of maturity I could claim once I reached optimal health. I had a wife and three kids to think about, though the things I used to worry would kill me — like hundreds of extra pounds — were now in the process of literally disappearing from my body. Getting life insurance, I figured, was going to be a piece of cake.

The day came when I found myself on the phone with a life insurance representative who was running through what he assured me were boilerplate pre-screening questions. *What was my current age? How tall was I? How much did I weigh? Was I married? How many children did I have? What did I do for a living? Did I smoke?* When he asked how much alcohol I drank, I was able to answer, firmly: "I don't drink alcohol. At all."

"And what is your waist size?" he asked.

Thinking back on those coffin-drapery sized, fifty-four-inch-waist pants that tormented me from the end of the bed months before, I said, proudly, "Forty."

There was a pause. I heard the leafing through of pages and the clicking of a pen. "And your height again, Mr. Stewart?"

"Five-foot-nine. Is there a problem?"

"Well, Mr. Stewart, that means you are morbidly obese."

"What are you talking about? I'm five-foot-nine, I weigh two-hundred and forty pounds, and I have a forty-inch waist. I am not *morbidly obese.*"

"According to the numbers you gave me, Mr. Stewart, yes — you are severely overweight. We would like to see a waist size of thirty-two inches on men of your height."

"Look, I know my dimensions aren't *standard fare,*" I said, wag-gishly, "but I run over sixty kilometres per week. Last week, I ran a sub-thirty-minute 5K —"

"Mr. Stewart, I am sorry, but you are not eligible for life insur-ance at your current size. You need to take another eight inches, *minimum,* off your waist size."

"How is this more about my waist size than my weight?"

"We have to be very careful about who we provide coverage to, Mr. Stewart. I'm sure you can appreciate that."

"Look, can I send you a photo? So you can see that I am not morbidly obese —"

"I'm sorry, Mr. Stewart, there is no point in continuing with the screening. Have a nice day."

I stood there, staring blankly out our front door. It was an un-seasonably warm spring day, and the street steamed in the humid afterglow of an afternoon thunderstorm that had just rolled through. I snapped my fingers next to my ear. There was a high, insectile whine deep in my head, but everything else sounded far away, underwater. There was either a swarm of cicadas or a tornado cell descending on the neighbourhood, or my discussion with the insurance screener had sent my blood pressure through the roof.

It was broad daylight. It was supposed to be a day off from running ... but there was going to be a change of schedule, and routine.

"Who was that?" It was Jennifer at my elbow.

"Nobody. A guy from the life insurance company."

"Which was it," she laughed. "Nobody or somebody about life insurance?"

"Both. I'm going for a run."

○　○　○

In the nearly five months since my double circuit of Willistead Park, I had stripped nearly ninety pounds from my body. I had committed myself to lose one hundred pounds before my fortieth birthday. That was still over a year away. Running was transforming me. It was like a terraforming operation happening all across my body: shapes and sizes were obviously changing, and things I hadn't known were even there — things like ribs, joints, and other bones — were becoming visible.

The size and shape of my feet actually changed; shoes I'd purchased six months previous were now too large, particularly in the width, because without ninety extra pounds pushing down on them all day, my feet had become narrower. My hands looked lean, veiny, and strong, instead of puffy and sausage-like. My wedding band had to be resized in order to keep it on my hand, but, thanks to running, it was a short-lived fix — additional weight loss required me to retire the band to Jennifer's jewellery box because repeated resizing was going to ruin the integrity of the gold.

My armpits became hollows rather than protuberances. I could see my own genitalia, which, much to the delight of everyone involved (Jennifer and I) was emerging from the receding glacier of my flesh, appearing larger and experiencing much better blood flow. My stomach skin, once tight as a drum, was now a slack fold of excess flesh and scar tissue.

Inherently modest, it's not like I was aching to run around town without a shirt or cut the lawn in just my running shorts, but the fact that I wasn't actively shopping around for cut-rate cosmetic surgery showed that I was putting aside some of my self-conscious vanity. As I shrank and became denser and more compact, I was growing emotionally and psychologically.

But outside of all these small triumphs of the flesh — the visible, tangible, positive effects running had on my corporeal self — I came to realize that the real blessing of running transcends the physical.

Where walking had revealed to me the benefits of visual stimulation and the effects of slowly but continuously changing scenery on the imagination, running was taking that effect and picking up the pace to a point where I wasn't consciously thinking of anything. Running freed me up to *intuit* things. A habitual overthinker, I found myself finishing a run having little in my head except for visual and emotional memories that were completely disconnected from any concrete lines of thinking. It was a revelation, and a relief.

With the growing need to run came an increased awareness of how my body and mind reacted to physical activity. There are obvious, well-documented scientific reasons for this. Endorphins, for example, are known to work wonders for depression. I can attest to this. The more I ran, the more my mood stabilized. Problems — financial, work-related, family-related, writing-related — did not seem so overwhelming. In fact, nothing seemed overwhelming. If I ran 8 kilometres before heading into work at the newspaper, what part of my day was going to be more difficult, more strenuous, and more rewarding than that run? No part. Everything after the run was gravy. A very low-fat, high-fibre gravy.

I became more accepting and tolerant of situations, and at the same time, I became more intolerant of taking people's crap. I was not operating under the illusion that I was *in control*. In sobriety, I knew that the idea of my being in control of anything — wielding the toxic alcoholic willpower — was laughable and dangerous.

Which is why in the immediate, ear-ringing aftermath of my conversation with the insurance screener, I knew I could either let it ruin my day — sleep it off in a cocoon of embarrassment and revenge fantasy on the napping couch in my office, then wake up and, like a bear awaking from hibernation, rip into a box of cereal and sit on the kitchen floor dumping it down my throat ... or I could partake in the solution to my problem.

When I weighed nearly four hundred pounds, any negative interaction I had with another person resulted in me figuring I deserved to be treated poorly. Indulging in a different kind of masochism, I whipped myself with self-loathing, and the only salve for the raw wounds was food — my gluttony and shame supported each other. Now, although I was shrinking, with every pound I dropped, there was a corresponding uptick in the amount of confidence I gained. For the first time in years, I felt capable of defending myself, both physically and verbally. As much as the biases that made it impossible for me to qualify for affordable life insurance under any conventionally available policy chafed like a hair shirt on a long, hot run, the fact that I felt more capable of defending myself, and the fact that I was trying to live differently in sobriety not only prevented me, but relieved me, of the sense that I had to react; that I had to educate or change my doubters and detractors ... or hurt them — emotionally or physically. As much as I disliked body-shamers of every stripe, I tolerated them. Because as tough as it had always been for me to deal with people, the person I have always had the most antipathy toward and the least acceptance and tolerance of was *me*. Running, this physical activity, this sport, had provided grounds upon which I could accept my imperfections, and the imperfections of others. Running provided me with a way to avoid giving in to the most base and violent parts of my nature; a way to rise above the easy taunts and my own immature reactions. Running became my form of meditation.

Meditation is a very strongly suggested component of solid, long-term sobriety, and in my early days of recovery, I was very concerned with doing it right. As it turns out, my idea of what constitutes meditation was just as rigid and narrow as some people's idea of what constitutes a runner. I would remove myself to my home office and sit in my La-Z-Boy recliner, burn some incense, and try to empty my head of all thought. Sometime later, I would wake up with drool running down my chin and pooling on my chest. I continued on this way for several months, talking a big game about my meditative practice when all I was really doing was napping in a cloud of frankincense. Even though I knew its importance, meditation was not part of my sobriety until I started running. And with meditation, much like with sobriety, it was about progress, not perfection.

It was my initial obsession with the cold, hard data of running that allowed me to eventually see beyond the tangible, beyond the linear distances run, beyond the time and space coordinates and preoccupations with pace and max heart rate that filled my running app (linked by GPS to a satellite orbiting the Earth) as I set new Personal Bests and achieved various milestones. I would pore over my average pace times, top speed, split times, overall time, total calories burned, and, of course, the GPS map of every single run, so I could relive my routes from high above, or from street level.

But after a while, I realized something strange about my preoccupation with the run data, particularly when it came to the maps. I wasn't looking at them so much to relive or to remember the run — the neighbourhoods I'd run through; the landmarks

I'd passed — but rather to find out where I'd been; to see the run, sometimes, seemingly, for the first time.

Musing on this meditative state in my running journal, I wrote the following: "When I'm running, I am somewhere else. Not just as far as the geographical points plotted on a GPS map ... but interiorly. It's like I am somewhere inside myself." It took me a few days to figure out where I'd come across this concept of *a place within the self* before; the notion that writers and artists are always looking for hiding spots, real places that exist in the imagination as a place to survive. It was while showering after a run — anything particularly creative that has formulated in the depths of my head during the run usually bubbles to the surface in the shower — that I recalled the source: the eminent French philosopher, historian, and literary critic Michel Foucault's 1967 essay, "Of Other Spaces: Utopias and Heterotopias."

Foucault characterizes heterotopias as "a sort of simultaneously mythic and real contestation of the space in which we live ... privileged or sacred or forbidden places, *reserved for individuals who are, in relation to society and to the human environment in which they live, in a state of crisis*" (italics mine). Now, Foucault mentions adolescents, menstruating women, and the elderly as prime examples of those seeking heterotopias as a refuge from crisis. But everyone reaches their own bottom, and given the general acceptance of teens, menstruating women, and old people in present-day Canada, I am going to add sober alcoholic runners who have found a place of meditative serenity where they can survive, freed of the spectre of their obesity and their obsessive self-consciousness and self-loathing.

When I was running, I was elsewhere. On the map, but not *of* the map. I felt like I was away. Citing Galileo, Foucault backs me up on this idea that feeling it is necessary to be fixed in place is an old-fashioned concept: "This space of emplacement," Foucault writes "was opened up by Galileo. For the real scandal of Galileo's work lay not so much in his discovery, or rediscovery, that the Earth revolved around the sun, but in his constitution of an infinite, and infinitely open, space. In such a space, the place of the Middle Ages turned out to be dissolved, as it were; *a thing's place was no longer anything but a point in its movement, just as the stability of a thing was only its movement indefinitely slowed down*" (italics mine). Yes, I could look at my runs plotted out as GPS points on my laptop screen, but what was happening on that run, the great, life-altering benefit of the physical activity, for which the map served as a physical representation, was emotional, happening in my imagination, in a place that cannot be pinpointed on a map, or measured by time.

I never felt high in a drunk or stoned sense, but this blankness, this cessation of my tendency to over-analyze myself, my thoughts, my surroundings, and other people, was remarkable in its novelty and refreshing it its mindlessness. After years of not running because of fear, running had become a place I was consciously seeking, a refuge where I could go and abandon myself. This spiritual transformation, this wholesale change in my thinking — moving from a place of deep shame and self-loathing to one of acceptance and understanding — came from the meditative, calming, other-placeness of running. This is the best reason I can come up with for why my first year of running passed by with very little associated memory of running itself: it was meditative to the point where I was falling in love with that *out-of-mindness* that allowed me to run worry- and injury-free.

Foucault's beguiling theory on heterotopias certainly bore weight in my situation, but even with his overtures to the imagination and escapism, they were lacking something. I really didn't feel like I was escaping something so much as I felt like I was finally filling in that final piece of the hole that I used to fill up with booze and food, bringing all of myself to that spiritual malady that I could only comprehend or find or service in that ulterior space. I was surviving in those spaces — thriving even — but finding a way to talk about them was eluding me.

It wasn't until I began writing this book that I realized what it was. Tasked with coming up with a cool title, I started a list in my running notebook. The list grew to precisely three entries:

RUNNING IS AN IMAGINARY PLACE IN MY HEAD
THE RUNNING-SHAPED VACUUM
THE RUNNING-SHAPED HOLE

The vacuum concept that had reminded me of something Martin Deck, Windsor's pre-eminent bookseller, had said to me following a regrettable social media conflagration that erupted in the CanLit scene upon the death of noted critic and celebrity atheist Christopher Hitchens. A well-known Toronto-based literary pundit had posted a link to a news item about Hitchens's death and had invited everyone to reply with a comment detailing the most important thing Hitchens had taught them. I posted that the most important thing Hitchens had taught me was that it is possible to be a brilliant literary critic while simultaneously having no clue what you are talking about on the subject of God, faith, and spirituality. The backlash was quick, severe, and comical. I lost friends. People openly renounced my poetry. Commiserating with me via private message about how many people involved in the online brawl reacted — much like Hitchens himself — in anger and fear at any mention of God or faith, Martin said, "They don't recognize the God-shaped hole is God-shaped."

It matters very little to me that this was Martin paraphrasing Pascal because I would never have recognized this as Pascal. I came to this concept of the God-shaped hole and its bastardization to "running-shaped hole" through Martin Deck, and I am giving him full credit. I had written it down in a totally different, non-running-related notebook at the time, thinking it was something he had uttered in his natural profundity.

When it occurred to me, though, that it could serve as a possible book title, I went leafing back through two years of notebooks to December 2011 and the whole sordid Hitchens affair (more than fourteen months before I took my first steps as a committed runner) and immediately queried Martin on what he had said. He pointed me to Pascal's *Pensées*.

In Section X, "The Sovereign Good," Pascal argues that all of humanity seeks happiness, but we lack the ability to attain it for ourselves and attempt, instead, to fill the vacuum, or void, with the kind of worldly, wanton things that fallen, imperfect humans want. We always believe our expectations will be met this time, failing to remember that the things we think will make us happy have only led us toward disappointment time and time again. "So, while the present never satisfies us, experience deceives us," Pascal writes, "and leads us from one misfortune to another until death comes as the ultimate and external climax."

We do this because we fail to recognize, over and over again, that what we really want is a relationship with God, a more spiritual existence. We fail to see, as Martin Deck explained so succinctly, that even when we are crying out in anguish and grief, seeking to understand and be understood, that the void we are seeking to fill is God-shaped. In failing to recognize this, and in failing to recognize God's necessary and rightful place in that hole, says Pascal, humanity "can know neither true good nor justice."

What kind of person can fill the God-shaped hole and still have a running-shaped hole to fill? Probably an alcoholic. But it is not God's failing. It is His gift. He left something else for me to find, something that would make me surrender the defect that kept my eating out of control and my body morbidly overweight. *A running-shaped hole.* Just as I had with sobriety, I had to get there on my own. No one could lead me there. The moment of clarity about food and my weight that I had had while leaving the cardiology appointment on November 28, 2012, was no different in quality or effect than the one I had with alcohol, standing in the Avalon Front in downtown Windsor on April 11, 2003.

Running was, and always had been, the missing puzzle piece, the thing that filled the ever-darkening, ever-widening void. It became the meditation I needed in order to improve my conscious contact with something greater than me: something greater than books and cameras; something greater than my career, music, movies, and baseball; something greater than any drug or drink, and, of course, something better than food.

The less poetic would say they are *in the pocket,* or *in a zone.* In the running community, it's called a *runner's high,* but the combination buzz of endorphins and heightened respiration is an acute and fleeting sensation and does not begin to touch the lasting fulfillment that running provides. The only thing I know that does that is a spiritual experience. Finding, occupying, and filling the running-shaped hole, for me, is just that: a spiritual experience. It makes me more tolerant and accepting of myself. It subdues my self-consciousness and self-loathing. I become more open to the contradictory nature of my character and find some measure of peace in the fact that progress, for me, isn't always a linear path toward immediate grace, generosity, and perfection. And if I am more at peace with myself, I feel I become — not in a purely physical, less corpulent way but on a positive psychic energy and happiness-exuding level — more acceptable to others.

So, it's a good thing running also works toward making me more tolerant and accepting of others because one of the things being overweight and unhealthy did was separate me from other people. Running makes room for them; running makes me want to fill loneliness with people, rather than with food consumed in isolation. Like many spiritual experiences, the running-shaped hole creates an outward expansiveness, a positive aspect, that, for me, does not come naturally; nor does it always show. But the more I run, the more I feel it and recognize it in how I think and act. If I can tolerate me, I can sure as hell tolerate you. Running, I realized fairly early on, was connecting me to people.

◦ ◦ ◦

As is often the case, the rain had done nothing to cool things down on this particular day, and as I stepped out onto the front porch after the insurance screener's phone call, I could feel the air in my mouth and chest. It had weight. The place was like a ghost town. Everyone was inside, hiding from the storm, however brief it had been, and the swampy heat that followed. There was a time when I would have been pleased to think they were hiding from me, hiding from my temper as it reached its peak ferocity in the tyrannically unhinged words I would have directed at the screener following the news of my being turned down for life insurance. My anger would have forced them to lay low, sheltering in place so as not to rile me further with their attempts at jocularity and overtures of friendship … But no longer. I didn't want to be that person anymore. And I wasn't about to let some box-checking, corporate-policy wonk control my day and how I felt about myself. I had a choice. I could choose to run. I could choose to run in broad daylight whenever I liked.

In running, I found the peace that the God of my understanding wants me to know. I had come to realize that avoiding the precipice of the running-shaped hole was not the object of running; there was no benefit to be had, no future to be gained, in skirting the void, in running away from anything. Running had led me, literally, to a pathway in an idyllic setting. I could either embrace the pathway humbly and quietly, or I could stray from it, indulging in all the worst parts of my character, revelling in the most depraved and vacuous kinds of social drama, turning my back on the hard-won knowledge that I had to maintain a certain spiritual condition — to stay focused on the pathways as a place to run and meditate — in order to be a sane, acceptable member of society. The true danger of the running-shaped hole is forgetting that there is a running-shaped hole, a spiritual emptiness that needs to be tended to on a daily basis. The point of the running-shaped hole, then, is to run toward it, to run in it, to occupy it wholly.

This is what I set out to find that sticky day — my bronzed and tattooed arms slick with sweat, the fiery-orange running singlet already stuck to my back before I even left the front porch — not to find some random life insurance screener on whom I could take out my indignant rage by forcing them to run with me. Surely, a life insurance screener must be of unimpeachable personal habits with the physiognomic specifications of a Sears catalogue model ...

"You will feel better after you run," Jennifer said, kissing my shoulder. "Don't take the guy on the phone with you. He doesn't know how sexy you are." That was all I needed to hear. I left the guy on the phone in a pile on the front porch.

Nearly every time I ran, I was able to find that space and occupy that space anew, by giving over my natural inclinations toward stasis and leisure, by getting uncomfortable. Running is not easy. If it were, everyone would be doing it.

CHAPTER SIX

MOON OVER THE SUPER-SOFT TARGET

AT THE SPRING Thaw 5K, I had picked up that registration form for the Running Factory's spring Learn to Run (LTR) Clinic. Other people, in groups, running next to me, at my pace — maybe with the same fears and particular biases and hatreds of self — could be exactly what I needed to push my running to the next level. Besides, my expansive new attitude was supposed to be repairing the chasm between me and other people! I filled out the LTR registration and took it, along with my $62 registration fee, to the Running Factory, several days in advance of the clinic's April 15 start date.

What was bound to be an auspicious day — the day I so selflessly took my burgeoning love of running and gave it to a community! — became decidedly more ominous when, just before 3:00 p.m., two pressure cookers full of nails, ball bearings, and black powder exploded near the finish line of the 117th running of the Boston

Marathon. Three people died. Sixteen people lost limbs. There was little doubt, even in the very early stages of the developing news story, that this was a terrorist attack.

Sitting in the Windsor-Essex Community Publishing editorial bullpen, we watched the newsfeeds, saw the photos, felt the chaos that the attack was intended to inflict. I had friends who were in Boston to run the marathon. Checking their Facebook pages, I saw that they were checking in as "Safe," (as journalists we were always, ghoulishly, searching for that local angle to any international tragedy). And even though Boston is 1,134 kilometres from Windsor, I am the kind of easily worried person who takes terrorism very personally. I saw how mundane the underpinnings of such an attack were (department store-grade pressure cookers, backpacks, crowds, large scale public events); I saw how easy it was to know someone who had, for a few minutes earlier in the day, been within the blast radius of the two explosions. Whether by dint of their running prowess or by sheer luck, my friends had finished their races and, likely exhausted, moved on from the Boylston Street finish line. This kind of happenstantial border between safety and victimhood was just too tenuous and porous for me not to feel personally affected. Terrorism works on me the way I suspect it works on most people: it terrifies.

It would have been easy to drive home from work that day, round up the children, lock the doors, and batten down the house against whatever extremist shitshow was about to shut down the continent. Yes, I'd already registered and paid for the Learn to Run Clinic. Yes, my running gear was already set out so I could make the easy transition from newspaper editor to runner, but this was an extenuating circumstance, possibly a matter of national security. It would have been all too easy to become transfixed by the lure of the news coverage of the bombing. When is television better than when the world is about to end? There would be hours of uninterrupted, hyper-intense speculation available on TV (not to mention a veritable bonanza of opinions, false flags, and conspiracies on social media). And although the media frenzy surrounding the bombing stoked the same kind of fears for my own well-being that the prospect of running used to inspire — death in all of its chaotic and inexplicable gruesomeness arriving swiftly and without mercy — I did not let the fears impede my decision to lace up and get out the door, arriving at the Running Factory in advance of the clinic's 6:15 p.m. start time.

Although by the spring of 2013, I was already running every other day and had lost about ninety pounds, my running was still plagued by fear: an existential dread that crept in, especially on longer runs. As my distances crept up into the 10- to 12-kilometre range and beyond, I would start to feel like the falcon who has flown so far afield that it can no longer hear the falconer. This untethered, off-the-grid feeling mirrored almost identically the bowel-churning separation anxiety I experienced as a child when I was allowed to walk down to a bookstore in the mall by myself while my parents did the grocery shopping. As much as the young me enjoyed this small, liberating measure of freedom and maturity such excursions afforded, the loneliness and desolation of the primal fear of being separated from my parents would overcome me like a slow-acting horror.

Similarly, while running, the anxiety didn't rise up to meet me like the road when you've toed a crack in the pavement, but, rather, it drifted lightly down, like gossamer: a creeping dread that manifested itself in my not wanting to admit that I am, somehow, for some reason, afraid. *I'm a grown man! I'm running in a city I've lived in my whole life! It's broad daylight! What am I afraid of?*

But rather than just admit that I was feeling lonely and afraid, I would try to recast this nebulous anxiety as something else. Maybe I was bored? Surely boredom is more acceptable than fear?

Bored with the same old streets and routes, bored with my obsessive thoughts, bored of the pain of endurance running. None of these things were manifestly true, though, when I stepped back and thought about it, especially given my professed love for the street-level view of the city running provided and the meditative clarity it brought to my mind.

But this meditation on the interplay between anxiety and boredom put me in mind of something my old friend and mentor, the poet and scholar Tom Dilworth, says, famously (at least around here): *boredom is horror spread thin.* Something of an artful intuition wrapped in an aphoristic quip, Tom's bon mot isn't a psychologically supported position, but it's always spoken to me on the deep level of poetry. I've always taken it to mean that the things that are present in horror that are monstrous and shocking are also present in boredom, just in a more diluted form. What appals us with boredom, though, is deprived of much of its macabre power because we experience it slowly, over time. Instead of being suddenly shocked by something appalling, I experience a kind of malaise or ennui, one inspired by a thing that I find difficult to identify.

The plasticity of time — its strange amplifications and attenuations — played a part in my struggles with alcohol and with curbing my out-of-control eating. Whereas my drinking produced sudden horrors and had an immediate and gut-wrenching impact on my family, my career, and my well-being, the horrors of overeating were experienced slowly, over a distended length of time. My morbid weight gain occurred in small increments. I was able to ignore it for a long time, then, suddenly, a well- (or poorly) timed family photo ripped the scales from my eyes. The toxic effects of my overeating and mounting obesity had taken on a languorous quality, inducing a state that was something akin to boredom, despite its having many striking similarities to the visceral and chaotic circumstances of my drinking, which were recalled with horror.

I spent a lot of time wondering which of these equally vexing states of boredom and anxiety I was encountering while running from my demons and came to this horrifically boring and angst-inspiring conclusion: maybe what I was experiencing *wasn't* the anxiety of being separated from my loved ones, or the anxiety, say, of failing to fulfill my domestic and professional obligations, or of failing to live up to other people's expectations, but was instead simply the stark boredom of being alone with myself.

My gut feeling is that almost anyone who has ever tried to adhere to a fitness routine will be familiar with using anxiety and boredom as excuses for prolonging stasis, with finding little justifications for why they shouldn't exercise today, or for the foreseeable future. But where most people would prefer not to follow these thoughts down the rabbit hole, pursuing the thoughts to their morbid ends, trying to figure out if they're actually bored or really just trying to talk themselves out of cycling, walking, deadlifting, or swimming, I am otherwise inclined. I am convinced that it all just comes down to the anxiety, the deep psychological horror of the prospect of being alone — actually or metaphorically out in the woods, where old, sick animals go to die in painful solitude.

◦ ◦ ◦

Such cheery thoughts took me back to that brief flirtation with Jennifer's LTR Duo-Tang some four years earlier — the flirtation that began with me standing on the sidewalk in front of our house, crying, and culminated in me twisting my ankle on the rutted Bruce Peninsula Road. Was I convinced I was going to keel over dead on a very light walk/run around the park, or was I just horrified by the vast expanse of loneliness I was confronted with, knowing that if my corporeal self held up, running may just bore me to death? And thinking of it, I was struck with a sudden insight:

the LTR Clinic, which featured one group run per week, was not so much designed to increase your 5K time as it was to increase a new runner's ability to combat the fear and boredom of running by fostering friendships through a supportive community. That's why I was here, on such a historically dreadful day … *to be part of.*

About sixty of us were gathered in the Running Factory's cramped retail space — a range of people of different ages, body types, and confidence levels, chatting nervously about the events unfolding in Boston. I'd been running four or five times per week, monitoring everything I ate and weighing myself every morning for more than six months. I felt lean and strong, but I also felt nervous about all the new faces and their unknown running abilities and unsettled by the bombings.

What if, I wondered (certainly not aloud to my fellow LTR participants), the Boston Marathon had been specifically targeted by terrorist organizations? What if it was the sport itself that had been selected for attack, selected because runners proudly indulge in an exuberant, mutually supportive, accepting lifestyle, and dress in colourful, form-fitting fashions (women included!), and do so largely in public view — all things that radical Islam hates? Post-9/11, everyone was aware of soft terrorist targets — shopping malls, sports arenas, hospitals, schools, movie theatres — but, in the Windsor-Essex Community Publishing editorial bullpen, my incorrigible colleagues and I had ruminated on super-soft targets, the kind of community events that populated the pages of our county-based weeklies: hayrides, orchard tours, bikini car washes, corn mazes, and pepper games. Low-stakes running group events certainly fit the bill. There had been four separate and coordinated hijackings on 9/11. What if today saw similarly coordinated attacks against running groups and clinics across North America? There were ample opportunities to stash IEDs in any number of municipal trash bins, bus kiosks, and garden planters around town.

You could run down a group of runners in a vehicle virtually anywhere along the route. An incendiary could be buried in the gutless void of the tech fibre–clad mannequin that stood next to the cash register in the Running Factory store at this very moment.

But no matter. I was living differently. I was not letting fear rule my thoughts; I was not allowing excuses to put me prostrate on the couch, insensate from overindulging in food — and I'd been living this way for a while. Finally, maybe, I was *wholly sober*. (Though clearly my thoughts could travel down some sick paths and entertain some seriously demented scenarios.)

Though new to the LTR Clinic, I was not entirely new to running, so when it came time to hit the pavement, I slotted myself in Group 4 — for more experienced runners who can run continuously for fifty-five minutes, want to improve their 5K times, or want to run a 10K — and we set out on our Week 1 group run.

The things I had always been so skeptical of — the fellowship and camaraderie of the running community — I came to appreciate. They seemed comforting and helped me to allay my self-conscious fear of being too heavy and too out of shape to run. My self-doubt was further diminished by the passing motorists who honked and waved and shouted encouragement from their vehicle windows as we ran in a pack down Riverside Drive. It was overwhelming. The eight of us running west on our out-and-back route all waved back. Old biases about running and jealousies of particular friends who were runners (all of which I now recognized as classic contempt before investigation) fell away.

I realized the people in the passing vehicles probably thought we had gathered together to run in solidarity with those in Boston. Every runner who was out running — and there were lots; we passed them and they offered thumbs-ups, high-fives, and friendly greetings — probably experienced something like this on that day, a day when runners and running were making headlines for all the wrong reasons. I was coming to understand this: runners — runners everywhere — support each other. Even people who don't run, have never been runners, recognize that runners do something kind of remarkable — definitely crazy, but also kind of remarkable.

It had not been the elite race leaders, the potential Olympians, and endorsement deal-wearing record setters of the running world who had been targeted that afternoon in Boston. It had been the middle-of-the-packers, the everyday runners who ran between shifts in the factory, on weekends, or on vacations while the rest of their families were eating funnel cake and laughing at foibles that will pass on into clan lore. Those were the people who were knocked to the ground by the blasts. It was their family members, lining Boylston Street to cheer on not just their kin, but anyone running the marathon, competing in one of the most iconic races and one of the most physically and emotionally demanding things a person can decide to undertake, who were ripped apart by the ball bearings and scrap metal in those pressure cookers. It was their blood that literally ran in the streets. And the running community — a community I was now, suddenly very much a part of — had been the target.

I realized that even if you are running alone, you are part of the running community. It is why runners — most runners — acknowledge each other on the streets, pathways, and trails, like boaters in cottage country. And I realized that if you participate in the sport of running, if you have access to the kind of uplifting, transformative power of running but are overly competitive, standoffish, arrogant, and unhelpful you may be a runner but you are also an asshole.

Running connected me to people and to a community in a way that went wholly against my natural inclination. Filling that running-shaped hole — a process that had started (can only start) as a solitary pursuit — had given me that rare thing: the feeling of being part of.

○ ○ ○

Although I was eventually asked to be a group leader in the Learn to Run Clinic, and even though I knew that participating in the clinic had made me more tolerant of others and had helped me see running as a larger community, any enjoyment I got out of the group running experience came from doing something in direct opposition to my instincts. If running was about pushing physical limitations and overcoming psychological barriers, I figured I might as well chafe against my antipathies toward group experiences while doing it.

Granted, the Learn to Run Clinics represent group running at its positively convivial best. I had heard tell of running groups that wore their exclusivity on their sleeves — literally, as they required members to wear flashy, group-branded singlets, tech hats, and warm-up suits — and kept their ranks closed and their competitive edges honed to a state of stand-offishness. This was the running community's worst aspect, its seedy, self-important underbelly, and I was loath to get involved in anything so pretentious. Strange, then, that I ended up in a second running group that took its exclusivity to extremes, turning closed ranks into a hermitic virtue.

I first met Kira Kovacs through the poetry community. We read together a few times in Toronto, and when the readings were done and our fellow poets wanted to talk about writing and other writers, we found ourselves talking about running. We ran together very infrequently, given that she lived in Toronto, but we would often text each other before, after, and even during training runs. And this communication was working for us, keeping us motivated as we watched each other's run stats climb through the weeks and months on the running app we both used.

The running group we formed was designed for two people who lived in different cities and rarely saw each other, who stood proudly and self-parodically unaffiliated with any other runners or groups — notwithstanding my clearly conflicted and self-conscious affiliation with the Learn to Run Clinic. Anyone accusing us of "hypocrisy" because of our membership restrictions was clearly discounting the fact that both Kira and I were poets, which ought to have been deterrence enough for almost anyone seeking membership. We discussed our resistance to giving the group a name and decided to avoid doing so, just to make it extra off-brand and against type. Indeed, the only stipulation for membership was that you had to end your long runs at an ice-cream parlour — and from that, our little group unfurled the self-deprecating banner under which we ran: an ice-cream cone became our symbol.

I imagined someone asking me, "Hey, what's the name of that little running group you're in?"

"Do you know what an ice-cream cone looks like?"

"Well, yes —"

"Well, that's the name of the running group," I would reply, before hitting START on my watch and taking off into the evening sun, in search of a double-scoop of tiger tail on a waffle cone.

Kira drew a large cone on an old tank top with a Sharpie and sent a photo; I had Nathanael draw one on my upper arm with a marker before an 18-kilometre training run. The route for this particular run was eastbound along the riverfront, then along the Ganatchio Trail (one of Windsor's major running arteries) and ending at Stop 26 ice-cream parlour on Riverside Drive East, near the border with the Town of Tecumseh, where Jennifer and the kids met me to eat ice cream on a trailside bench.

These four people were really the only group I needed, and they didn't have to run to be my biggest, oldest running support group — no fancy uniforms, no hard-sell insurance pitches … just four people in it for the long haul and since long before I took those first fearful steps.

And as we sat eating our ice creams in the evening sun as it disappeared behind the cicada drone, the bridge, and the Detroit skyline beyond, I knew I was ready for the next step in my running; that evening's run having served as a scouting mission for my next race: the Moon in June.

○   ○   ○

Held in the evening and contested over the city's Ganatchio and Little River Trail system, the Moon in June is Windsor's long-running summer 10K race and attracts runners from around southwestern Ontario. The day it was held, Jennifer was out of town at a weekend conference and the children were staying with her parents. My support group would be MIA for this one. Although I felt a bit lonely and anxious standing around the grass-covered lot behind the Riverside Sportsmen's Club waiting for the race to begin, I was able to put those feelings aside, somewhat, and turn my thoughts toward my training; toward the running-shaped hole, where I communed with my Higher Power and basked in the freedom from my thoughts. In a few minutes, when the gun went off, I would be able to get there.

I went into the race with a plan: find a comfortable pace, stick to it, don't get distracted by any run/walkers, focus on my own running, view only myself as the competition. Simple. And on that temperate June evening (there was no moon to speak of), it worked perfectly. I settled into my eight-minute-per-kilometre pace and crossed the finish line with a time of 1:19:49 — good for dead last, 175th of 175 registrants — three minutes behind the 174th-place finisher.

Of course, I didn't realize I was the last runner out on the course as I merged onto the soft grass behind the Riverside Sportsmen's Club and put the pedal to the metal for the final two hundred metres. But I wasn't worried about my place on the list of chip time results. Although I'd covered the distance many times in training, I was just thrilled to be charging down the chute, enough fuel left in the tank for a solid sprint to the finish line.

Waiting for me on the other side, cheering me on as I crossed, bringing the Moon in June to a close, were all the other LTR group leaders. They surrounded me in a mess of embraces, playful head-locks, and high-fives. My running community didn't care that I was dead last; in fact, they celebrated it.

"You ran your race," said Brad, thrilled for me. "You crossed the finish line upright and smiling, and you had quite a kick down the stretch. That means you ran it right — didn't go out too fast, had something to give at the end."

He was right. That was all that mattered right then and there, outside a big tent awash with the smell of barbecued hot dogs and sweaty runners. For that night, and for the days-long afterglow of the Moon in June, I was cool with group running.

CHAPTER SEVEN

WHITE WASP

I'M LYING IN the fetal position in our bed, covered with every blanket Jennifer could get her hands on, as well as all three kids and Mycroft the Lakeland terrier — all are piled up on top of me while I shiver uncontrollably, teeth chattering, feeling like I am going to vomit all over the apple Jen is holding to my mouth.

"You can't keep doing this," she says, bemused. "It scares the kids. And it can't be good for you."

She's right, of course. I know better. But I have nothing to say. No defence. I cannot speak. I am numb. I am passing out.

At some point, I will wake up alone in the bed, everyone including the dog having abandoned their posts once I've slipped into an exhausted oblivion, with a half-eaten apple on the pillow next to me. But this is no scene from my drunken years of active alcoholism. This is me, post-run, at the height of my running fervour, shivering in near hypothermic conditions under a household of linen, trying to absorb the body heat of four people and a dog. And if you pan out the bedroom window onto the street, the city is not suffering under a brutal polar vortex. Outside, there is bright sun, parched lawns, and the omnipresent threat of thunderstorms — the thick of an Essex County summer.

During July and August in Windsor and Essex County, the humidex rarely dips below 35°C, day or night. The challenge for local runners becomes, simply, breathing. Our air quality, due to heavy industrialization and the metropolitan population that includes Detroit and southeastern Michigan, is poor to begin with. Mix in the swampy air and the low elevation, and a stroll through the park becomes a workout.

My long runs had taken on an exhilarating element of *survival*. Even if I left home with what I thought was ample water, I was, more than once, left as you see me in the scene described: dehydrated, delirious, and physically depleted. At the end of almost any long run, the sodium extracted through my skin by profuse sweating would be encrusted on my face, neck, and my arms from shoulder to wrist. I glittered in the sun like a sequined gown.

But what was more likely to bring me down was the fact that once the salt reached a critical mass on the surface of my body, I would stop sweating all together and, very suddenly, become very ominously cool to the touch. When I stopped sweating, I was usually several kilometres from home. Sadly, by that point, though, it was usually too late. Even with a store-bought energy drink and some quick candy carbs — low blood sugar was obviously a problem, too; a typical long run would see me burn upwards of 1,500 calories — there was no way I could stem the depletion of my body's resources. The salt crash was coming: severe chills, tremors, dizziness, nausea, anxiety, the scene on the bed. With trembling hands, I would make the call to Jennifer, giving her my rescue coordinates.

There are a lot of things that scare me about running. But as unpleasant and acutely frightening as these salt crashes (as I came to call them) were, they did little to deter me from running.

My running achievements may have been modest in the grand scale of things, but pride prefers a grand scale over modesty. I knew that a lot of my early success as a runner (so capably exhibited in any of the near-death experiences outlined above) could be attributed to my refusal to cut myself any slack. I had cut myself all the slack I could handle over the years, and it had been ruinous. Running was hard work, and I was going to be equally hard on myself. Once I realized I could run 2 kilometres at a stretch (after running home from my friend's that rainy February night), walking became, for me, passé. A mature, reasonable runner will learn to take regular walk breaks, particularly in the punishing summer heat. But I was not yet either of those things. I would not allow myself this small reprieve during a run, in part because it underscored the reality that I was not actually an elite runner, nor infallible, but mostly because it reminded me of taking the easier, softer path.

As training methods go, this is, of course, not widely recommended. It's predicated on the kind of hubris capable of striking a person down on a running path on any given day; and given Windsor's propensity for humidex advisories and heat emergencies, I was particularly vulnerable in the summer. I was pushing what I knew wasn't so much my luck as the bounds of a blessing. But because nothing irreversibly bad had happened yet as the result of my obstinacy, I was willing to push it. There were no regrets behind me, just well-worn running shoes, a pile of sodden running clothes, and rapidly shed pounds. And, Jennifer reminded me, children who did not like seeing me enfeebled and crystalline on the bed, quaking like a buzz bomb beneath the collective weight of their little worried bodies.

"Thomasin worries more than the boys," Jennifer told me. "She watches out the window for you when you're out running. More than once she's asked if we can get in the van and go find you."

It was true. Our daughter's anxiety was becoming a problem. She was seven at the time, and the sleepless nights she spent worried that either Jennifer or I, or one of her brothers, was going to be struck down by disease would leave her exhausted and stressed out at school. We sought a referral for her to see a psychologist and received a diagnosis. Like anyone, Thomasin had good stretches and bad, but the sight of me crashed out as a result of the very activity that had returned me to health corresponded exactly to the kind of health-scare scenario that often found her weeping silently in bed in the middle of the night. The running, she feared, was going to take me out.

I would be lacing up my shoes, and she would launch into a verbal checklist of safety and equipment: "Papa," she had taken to calling me, "do you have your hat? Did you put on sunscreen? On your ears? Do you have your phone? It's charged? Do you have water? Do you have money in case something bad happens and you need more water?"

Too much thinking, living too much in my head, as Dr. Sijan had warned me, was going to make happiness elusive and difficult. So, she came by it naturally. I knew how it felt to worry like that. But before her eighth year, she was surpassing me, whereas I had found a solution, a solution that scared her because I seemed so heedless, so fearless. But it was a solution I could share with her one day if she would let me.

○ ○ ○

When my old friend James Grant, who placed fourteenth overall in the 2005 Seattle Marathon with a time of 2:50:08, came home to Windsor for a visit in September 2013, he suggested we go for a run along the banks of the Detroit River. Even for late summer, it was unseasonably hot and humid. I was nervous going into the run because I was going to be running with the person who was likely the most accomplished runner I knew. Someone who regularly trained with Olympians would surely look critically on my slow pace, my copious sweating, my amateurish need for water ... Of course, nothing of the sort happened. James, though clearly not challenged with my 7:48 pace, was just happy to be running with his old friend. He had long been one of my encouragers, having once urged me to come out for a pre-dawn group 10K in Ottawa the morning of his wedding, when I was tipping the scale at upwards of 350 pounds. His visit home to Windsor was my chance to put behind me the immobility and paralyzing fear of the past, when I had to decline his well-meaning invitation for fear of dropping dead in the streets of an unfamiliar town on his wedding day.

Partway through our run on that unseasonably humid September afternoon, James suggested we take a walk. I wasn't struggling. We were carrying on a normal running conversation between old friends — kids, family, work, books. There was no reason to slow to a walk then, other than the fact that, in James's experience, walk breaks are standard training procedure for the high-level, long-distance runner. We walked for a few hundred metres then we picked up the run again. We took another walk break and ran the last 1.5 kilometres to my front porch.

We were sitting there, drinking water, and cooling down, and all I could think was, *Yeah, it was great to run with Jamie, but I sure wish I had my "A" game with me today because then he wouldn't have suggested those walk breaks. He would know I'm a real runner and he wouldn't be sitting there thinking today's run was a bust.* It was unfair of me to allow my fear of being judged — a vestigial effect of my extreme self-consciousness of morbid obesity — to lead me into judging my friend, especially when he was genuinely thrilled that we had finally run together. The walk break, this time suggested by a near-pro, was ruining my perception of what had been a decent 8-kilometre run.

Every once in a while, I get to run with my "long-distance" training partner, Kira. She has been advised by her doctor to take regular walk breaks during her runs because of the beta blockers she takes for blood pressure issues. When I run with Kira, I take the walk break. I don't complain because that would be selfish and rude. I don't try to talk her out of it because that would be even more selfish, not to mention dangerous for her. We simply take the one- or two-minute walk break. To be honest, I wish I wasn't taking the walk breaks. It always seems like, somehow, my run is sullied, rendered incomplete by even the briefest period of walking. I can't stop myself from thinking that it reflects poorly on my effort. It messes up my time. For Kira, it's completely necessary, and I'm there to support her walking. For me, well, I'm only doing this for Kira.

When running alone, I afford myself no such compassion. The voice that told me to ease up on a run when my legs were full of exhaustion's sand and sweat dripped off the brim of my hat, was treated with suspicion, a chimera of my past idleness and dilatory ways, urging me to wreck myself on the rocks of bad pace, bad form, and bad run. And as I actively ignored the voices, I would think of the late Steve Prefontaine, the American track star and running quote-machine, and his amazing observation that you should "not [be] running to see who is fastest, but running to see who has the most guts." I knew that as cool as it was to align myself with the tragic figure of Pre, I should probably just forgive myself for the failings of the flesh, and ... no — I could hear the voice, I just needed to listen to the voice. I needed to find some way of focusing on the mindfulness and overarching meta-ness of running — how it enabled you to transcend the moment by staying firmly in the moment; to transcend pain by understanding that running is supposed to be precisely this difficult and painful.

And with those thoughts in mind, while running along the Ganatchio Trail one late-summer afternoon in forty-degree-plus heat and humidity on what I still consider the worst run of my running career, I finally broke down. I allowed myself to listen to what I had learned from others about running and training smart. Why? Because humidity, like alcohol, is a cunning, baffling, and powerful foe.

It doesn't cause me acute pain or ruin my form and throw off my stride. And while I enjoy a good full-body sweat, the mindless moment, the joy I find in the running-shaped hole, is lost one drop at a time, replaced by a plague of negative thoughts: the embarrassments of the past, worries about the future, and the attendant concerns and responsibilities of the day. It sucks the life right out of the run and fills me with ennui and despair.

On this particular day, I felt also a very real fear, as I realized that a man of my size, pushing himself in such inhospitable heat, could find himself crumpled up on the side of the road, needing to be rescued and/or resuscitated by a passerby or EMS. My breathing became restricted. And it wasn't something I could chalk up to Windsor's famously industrial, low-lying, poor air quality. This was the early manifestations of panic; fear cinched like a choke chain around my throat. Clearly, I was no Steve Prefontaine. The chances of my dropping my guts right there on the trail were greater than my ever proving that I had superior intestinal fortitude. I was choking on my own stubbornness and pride when all I really had to do was take my ego off the throttle and walk it out.

So, I did. Eight times. That 11.15-kilometre run took me 1:29:57. I was furious with myself when I got home. I was admonishing myself and trying to figure why I had wussed out so badly. Was it dietary deficiencies? Hydration issues? Fatigue? Inadequate stretching? Wind direction? Was I carrying bad psychic baggage? Why was I so weak? The more I thought about the chain of fear I had felt, the more I realized that it wasn't something to admonish myself for. It was, in fact, a truly spiritual coming-to. There had been no salt crash. No nausea, no shakes. No family scene of the hypothermic father on the bed. I had taken walk breaks unprompted. And I realized that though it might take some getting used to, it was growth.

There's a big difference in challenging yourself to be a better runner by pushing through the physical discomforts of running and being a stubborn jackass. And although I wasn't happy with my results that sweltering day, I did take some satisfaction in the fact that I had done something contrary to my instinct; something I had been resisting even though on a deeper, intuitive level I knew it was the right thing to do.

One of the lessons I learned in getting sober applied just as well with food: in order to get well, I had to get uncomfortable. I had to allow myself to be a forty-year-old husband and father of three who used to weigh closer to four hundred pounds than two hundred pounds, who started running late in life and has a great deal to learn as a runner. Despite all the unspoken fear and physical pain resulting from my being sedentary and obese, it was allowing myself to be openly afraid of being powerless over food, and my unmistakeable obesity, that was truly uncomfortable for me. A born hypochondriac, I had always been convinced that my minor ailments, aches, and pains were harbingers of something much more serious and, of course, mercilessly fatal. This new, reasonable and measured approach to thinking about my health and what, on the surface, might look like sudden and unexplained tremors and confusion and exhaustion, was a sign of maturity — a maturity that began in sobriety but was honed on the hot, humid, and unwaveringly flat streets of Windsor. And on that day of that horrible, eight-walk-break-marred run, I matured as a runner, and as a person, because I had been open to running with others, and I had become willing to listen to what they said.

If I was finally willing to allow myself a mid-run break, I figured I might as well have something on hand to replenish my sodium levels while I was taking it because walk breaks alone would not protect me from a salt crash. I knew what the problem was, and I knew that there was a solution: better hydration combined with more sodium and electrolytes. There was a need, though, for prudence and caution: too much sodium and I felt simultaneously bloated and desiccated; too little, and my body could not properly regulate it temperature. I needed to strike a delicate balance and put an end to the salt crashes. They worried Jennifer and the children. They seemed to be a trigger for Thomasin's increased anxiety levels. And despite the simple biochemical explanation for them, explanations that even an English major could understand, when they happened, they were capable of making me think I was having a stroke or heart attack. And ruminating on whether or not I was having either of those rather serious medical complications — two of the very things I started running to avoid — was a recipe for a panic attack.

There's lots of science behind sports hydration and nutrition, but all you really need to know is that food gives your muscles energy to burn, and sodium and electrolytes help control hydration and body temperature and prevent muscle cramping. My research into the solution for the problem of salt crashes consisted of reading the product reviews in running magazines and talking to other runners, and then amassing, what, for a few months in the summer of 2013, was probably the largest private stockpile of running supplements in the continental Midwest.

There was the standard complement of energy gels, gummies, jelly beans, and lozenges; bottles of horse pill–sized electrolyte gel caps that looked like they held nothing but Peruvian marching power; and old-fashioned apothecary-style salt tablets that the guys in the auto plants and road crews popped like candy. I would pop a capsule before a run on a particularly hot, humid day and keep a stash of electrolyte edibles in my hydration belt to be administered as needed. I would mix and match products, looking for that optimal sodium threshold. And just like that — with just a few extra dashes of sodium in my run diet — the salt crashes went away.

But I had won the battle, not the war. Electrolyte supplements can be hard on the stomach, and soon I was running around with cellophane-wrapped discs of dehydrated raw ginger — good for settling the guts — to ward off vicious waves of stomach cramps and nausea. The ginger inevitably became a useless sticky mess in the pockets of my running shorts after removing the first piece. Add a clutch of Gu gels — filled with carbohydrates, protein, caffeine, and, usually, small doses of sodium — to the mess in my pockets and I was quickly feeling overburdened with hydration and energy supplements. Why couldn't they all just be one thing?

Listening to me stand in the kitchen and complain about this yet again, Jennifer, sick of my running supplement war chest/candied ginger cache infringing on our limited counter space, said, "Why don't you just make it all one thing?"

"Like, mash it all up into a golem or something?" I said, incredulous.

"Aside from being ridiculously expensive," she said, gesturing at my horded goodies, "they all do pretty much the same thing. And I've looked at the active ingredients — sodium, carbohydrates, protein, amino acids, caffeine … It's all stuff we have right here. You don't have to spend hundreds of dollars on this stuff. We can get one of those juice decanters with a spigot and keep it on a shelf in the fridge, and before you go for a run, you can fill your water bottle from there. And you can use fresh ginger …"

Thus began my quest to create my own sports drink: a single-medium energy and hydration source that would deliver sodium, electrolytes, and carbohydrates while calming the guts and quenching thirst.

Please know that what I concocted is by no means certified by health officials, nor proven by scientists to be effective, or, even tasty. The ingredients are literally what I found around our kitchen that day, and if you don't have a drink dispenser, you can make it right in your water bottle, or in a juice decanter, a mason jar — whatever's handy — eyeballing the ingredients accordingly: water (obvious benefit to runners); freshly squeezed lemons (thirst quenching, flavour); ginger — frozen, peeled, and zested (soothes the stomach); table salt (electrolytes, aids hydration); pure maple syrup (carbohydrates).

After concocting this for the first time, there I was, in a pair of running shorts and an old plaid shirt, standing in the middle of my kitchen holding a six-litre drink dispenser with a spigot that, with some rearranging of the shelves, slides neatly into the refrigerator. I filled a glass and took it out on the front porch in case I needed to spit it into the garden. I was immediately set upon by a swarm of wasps. I took a sip and set the glass down on the newel post. The wasps droned around the glass's sweaty rim. They knew quality when it was presented to them. They dug its cloudy-white, salty sweetness, its slightly pulpy, sour spiciness. I called it White Wasp in their honour.

Watching me fill my water bottle from the spigot before a run, Thomasin said, "How does that stop you from getting sick after your runs?"

"Well, it's magic. I found the recipe in an old book about running. Do you want to try it?"

"What's it taste like?"

"Well, do you like lemon-filled doughnuts? And syrup on your pancakes? And salty French fries? Ginger snaps?" She looked dubious, but when I asked if she wanted to try some, she nodded. I filled a small tumbler for her. As she was reaching for it, I pulled it back. "Wait — you're not allergic to water, are you?"

She laughed. "Papa, stop!"

The first sip made her cough. But standing there in the kitchen, she soldiered on and drank it.

"I know it doesn't taste that great," I said, "but it's an ancient runner's recipe, and it's preventing me from getting sick."

"I can feel it working," she said, patting her tummy. I kissed her on the head, and as I headed for the door, she said "I love you, Papa. Be safe." That was all. She knew I was protected under the auspices of magic.

I was halfway down the sidewalk, tinkering with my watch when Thomasin stuck her head out the door and called. "Wait, Papa — does it really have bumblebee pee in it?"

"No, honey. Who —"

"Then why do you call it Bee Piss?"

"I don't, honey. It's called White Wasp."

I could hear her brothers' cackling from all the way down at the road.

"White Wasp, riiiiight." She snapped her fingers and pointed at me. "Have a good run," she said and ducked back into the house.

Good old White Wasp. It's become a hot weather staple, and fresh batches with varying flavour profiles and degrees of potability appeared in the refrigerator through the high summer, when wasps and runners are at their craziest.

CHAPTER EIGHT

THE ME PRESS HALFER

ON OCTOBER 19, 2013, I posted the following on Facebook:

RUNNERS: Did you train for the Free Press Half-Marathon and fail to land a bib? Worried all your training, as great as it has been, is going to amount to nothing but a pile of sweaty running clothes and empty Gu packets on the laundry room floor? Want to go for a long run tomorrow (Sunday, Oct. 20) to celebrate all your hard work? Maybe even 21.1K worth? I'm going to leave the parking lot at Willistead Park at 2:00 p.m. If you're there, we run together. Pass this along to anyone who might be interested.

"I can't be the only one," I said to Jennifer, who stood over my shoulder.

"If you post it, they will come," she said, hopefully. "What do they say — if this many people say they are coming to your event on Facebook, it means *x* number of people will actually show up?"

"Sounds like you've really delved into the numbers," I said, archly.

She smacked me across the back of the head with a dish towel.

"I just don't want to do this alone."

"But you like running alone."

"This is different," I said. "I've never run this far before. It seems like something you shouldn't do alone."

"If I was running, I would do it with you."

I knew she meant it, felt bad about sabotaging her past running ambitions, and gave her a hug.

One person "liked" my post. Another commended my moxie. But that was all the action my post got. At some point the next morning, I re-posted my call to run with an "I'm serious. 2:00 p.m." tacked on. And at 2:00 p.m., I stood in the parking lot in Willistead Park, utterly alone. I'd failed to inspire anyone — including members of my own family — to run.

It was a crisp fall day, bright and still. The thirty-fifth running of the Detroit Free Press Marathon and Half-Marathon had been contested through the streets of Detroit and Windsor earlier that morning. One of the only international marathons in the world, it requires runners to cross into Windsor via the Ambassador Bridge and cross back into Detroit roughly 5 kilometres later at the Windsor-Detroit Tunnel. Some twenty-seven thousand runners had set out from the starting line on Fort Street in downtown Detroit before dawn. I was not one of them. Which is why all of this was necessary.

By 2:00 p.m. it was clear that "all of this" was just going to be *all of me*, as I was still standing all alone in the Willistead Park parking lot. I could either let loneliness take me out before the starting line, or I could accept what I had known for a long time: running, like my other preoccupation, writing, is ultimately a lonely undertaking, and it works best if I just embrace the solitary pursuit head-on. With my hydration belt weighted down with Gu gels and a full bottle of White Wasp, I exited the park through its stately main gates and headed east on Niagara Street to Walker Road. I wanted to make sure my route included some hills — of which there are scant few in Windsor and Essex County — so I swung right onto Wyandotte Street East and headed toward the CN Rail viaduct — a trestle bridge over a canyon-like four-way intersection at Drouillard Road; the kind of place local parents warn their children about when it comes to playing or riding their bikes. There are sidewalks for pedestrians, but the traffic on Wyandotte tends to race past, disconcertingly close. Not my favourite place to run, but bridges and hills figured heavily in today's mission. I was determined to get my fill.

A few short weeks before, I had been training — training with a zeal I had not trained with before, or since — to run the first leg of the Detroit Free Press Marathon Relay. Shiva Koushik, a founding member of the LaSalle Rotary Club and one of my most stalwart newspaper contacts in my job as the editor of the *LaSalle Post*, had called and conscripted me to run for his team — the eponymously dubbed Team Koushik.

It was one of the nicest phone calls I have ever received — certainly the nicest received at my desk at the newspaper, where it was often just constant criticism and vitriol from the readership. Team meetings were planned. Registration papers would be disseminated. I would not let Team Koushik down!

Shiva and his wife, Aruna, were always going out of their way to do nice things for me, often dropping off Indian delicacies and sweets at my desk along with useful community news tips. I had done numerous stories on their selfless exploits in their native India, where they, along with thousands of other Rotarians, inoculated countless children against polio. In 2011, long before any running or weight loss, the Koushiks returned from one of their inoculation missions to India with a beautiful kurta — a traditional Indian garment for men, comprised of a long-sleeved, Nehru-collared shirt that hangs down to the knee, worn over a pair of pants that are loose at the thighs and taper to the ankle. A pale champagne colour with a glittery thread woven through, this kurta was custom-tailored from material hand selected by Aruna in India and gifted to me upon their return to their home in LaSalle.

The whole point of the kurta was that I would be able to wear it to the LaSalle Rotary Club's India-themed Crystal Drop Gala in the winter of 2012. Aruna, unbeknownst to me, had eyeballed my dimensions for the kurta ... and had come up embarrassingly short (and, in places, comically wide) of the mark. The kurta shirt was on the verge of ripping apart when I tried it on. The sleeves squeezed my arms like sausage casings, the cuffs hung several inches beyond the tips of my fingers; the pants legs eclipsed the tips of my toes and lay unfurled on the carpet before me. I felt ponderous and misshapen; I felt bad for being so overweight and short that I could not properly model the gift of the Koushiks' generosity.

Aruna was dying to see me in the kurta in advance of the gala, wanting to make sure it didn't need to be taken in or let out anywhere, small alterations she was prepared to undertake herself. She called me several times, but I always found some excuse as to why I couldn't get to their home with the kurta for a proper fitting. Finally, no fool, Aruna asked me straight up: "Bob, tell me — is something wrong with the kurta? Does it not fit?" I could not lie to her any longer.

"I didn't want to say anything, it was such a nice and generous gift — but it's too small," I confessed. "And in some places too big, if that makes any sense."

"Bob, you must bring it to me immediately," she insisted. "They always leave one or two inches of material on the inside of the seam. We have room to play."

But I had already checked. There were a scant few millimetres of material on either side of the seams inside the kurta. And the pants were going to need hemming to the point of losing their intended shape. I brought the kurta to Aruna nonetheless. I was embarrassed and felt like an ingrate, which I wasn't, and a rapacious glutton, which I most certainly was. Aruna consoled me. They were going back to India again in a year's time. She would measure me and return with a kurta that fit.

Not if I could help it. The spectre of that diaphanous, champagne-coloured kurta, folded so neatly, so uselessly on a shelf in our bedroom closet before I turned it over, shame-faced, to Aruna, was a slow-burning but contributing factor in the weight loss that was to come. There was no way I was giving anyone my true gargantuan measurements — my waist size at the time was a 54 — to take to a poverty-stricken country were untold millions lived with the very real spectre of starvation on a daily basis. I would rather spurn the generosity of friends; make them feel guilty and ashamed for having forced ill-fitting clothes on me. I would rather go kurta-less into whatever future I was to have.

○   ○   ○

Wrapped up in my newfound love of running, I had leapt at the opportunity to participate in the relay as part of Shiva's team. The relay can be run by as few as two and as many as five runners. The plan for the five members of Team Koushik was that I would run the first 10-kilometre leg, getting us over the Ambassador Bridge and into Windsor then pass the baton to Shiva along Riverside Drive in front of the Art Gallery of Windsor. Shiva would then run the second 10-kilometre leg, through the Windsor-Detroit Tunnel and back into Detroit, where he would pass the baton over to the first of two runners who would cover the two short relay legs (5 kilometres each). Whoever was anchoring Team Koushik would run the fifth and final leg of 10 kilometres.

This was my first big training goal, and the Marathon Relay was a great way to ease myself into the running of a half-marathon, and eventually a full.

I immediately took to the running trails at Malden Park, a former landfill site in southwest Windsor. If I was going to get up and over the steep grade of the Ambassador Bridge in good time — frankly, I was seriously worried about being able to do it at all (while also being concerned about the Ambassador Bridge being listed as one of the primary terrorist targets in Canada and the U.S.) — I was going to have to log some kilometres on some hills. Malden Park offered the perfect opportunity for this; it boasts a large, multi-peaked hill criss-crossed by running trails. Windsor's highest point, it is a surprisingly verdant mountain despite it's be-ing, in essence, a pile of garbage over which a thin layer of topsoil has been spread, and it features one particularly steep climb on its northwest face: a narrow, gravel path that climbs about forty metres over its two-hundred-metre traverse — an incline the running com-munity calls Big Bertha.

Hill repeats help with cardio conditioning and endurance, ob-viously, but they also pay big dividends when it comes to running form and speed. I ran hill repeats on Big Bertha until she no longer seemed like much of an incline at all, and I waited for the call from Shiva about the Team Koushik meet-and-greet. Other than Shiva, I didn't know anyone on the team, but we would be forever bound by our triumphant 42.2K relay. When I finally did meet them, I wanted to present as a serious runner who was up to the task of the first leg of the relay.

But I never met the other three runners on our team.

About three weeks out from the relay, I received an email from Shiva. It was addressed to everyone on Team Koushik. Shiva informed us, with regret and embarrassment, that we would not be participating in the race because he had failed to register the team. Before there was even a Team Koushik, Shiva had attended an information session. He thought he was registering the team when he put his contact information down on a sheet of paper. But all he was doing was requesting more information. He got all the information about the various relay legs, team transportation to the finish line, required ID for border crossings … and he passed it all along dutifully. But we were just never in the running, and the registration window had closed very firmly some weeks before.

I was disappointed, and a bit incredulous, but I wasn't upset. Running had soothed that part of me that, a year previous, would have slammed something down on my desk in a rage, shouted some profanity at no one in particular, and gone to bed immediately upon arriving home from work. There's a term for this: a temper tantrum. In the past, I would have indulged in one and then followed it by a good sulk. But training to run over the Ambassador Bridge had introduced me to Malden Park and had elevated my running to a new level. Team Koushik was dead, but my running was on an upward trajectory.

Other runners began putting it in my head that I should see if I could register and run the Detroit Half myself. It seemed crazy, but the kind of crazy that runners like. My long-run distance was regularly between 10 and 14 kilometres, and I had heard that old running chestnut that on any given day a runner can double the distance of their longest run. The results wouldn't be pretty. There was high likelihood the runner may barf all over themselves and go cataleptic at the end ... But it can be done. It's called *gutting it out*. And I was all about gutting it out. I'd had enough of waiting for change. I'd found strength and courage in flat-out forcing it.

I began investigating the possibility of a bib transfer — for a fee, the race committee will transfer a bib purchased by a runner who, for whatever reason, cannot run the race to someone who wants to run and missed the official registration period. A friend's daughter had injured herself training for the Detroit Half and was selling her bib. But with less than two weeks to go before race day, the bib transfer window had closed.

There were also people who were urging me just to buy her bib and run *as her* — Stephanie Lyons, a woman in her twenties. The results would be posted under her name in perpetuity. I thought about it for all of five minutes and decided against it. Even though this wasn't banditing — the loathsome practice of running road races without paying or registering — as not only was the bib already paid for, but I would also pay the original race registrant for the opportunity to wear the bib, it just seemed like bad karma to run the race as someone else. With all the border security measures in place, it also seemed like a good way to end up in a Homeland Security black site. It also seemed like my Higher Power was trying to tell me something: I wasn't meant to run the Detroit Free Press Marathon Relay or Half-Marathon in 2013.

I tried to put it out of my mind. I told myself that I was happy just to be running. That I was proud of myself for having trained and for being prepared to run. I should have been satisfied with these gains. But I was not. A strange thought began to work away in my avid runner's brain: was it possible I could run my own version of the Detroit Free Press Half-Marathon?

It was that pride — that zeal for running; that growing infatuation with the running-shaped hole — that saw me put out that Facebook call for fellow runners who wanted to run a half-marathon distance; that found me standing there, alone, double checking my watch and the double knots in my laces at the appointed hour, waiting for what I hoped — *expected, prayed?* — would be at least one or two other runners to arrive.

○ ○ ○

About 4 kilometres into my run, I ran past the now-shuttered coffee chain where for about eight years I had met, two nights a week, with about forty sober friends. The McDonald's where we relocated our coffee klatch to is also on Wyandotte, as is the weird little bakery that used to sell cigarettes and keep the members of Elephant wreathed in smokes when our practice space had been in John's parents' basement, two blocks south. I ran past a five-pin bowling alley I had been kicked out of one afternoon after day-drinking with high-school friends, the owners having made the mistake of renting us a lane at the same time as a children's birthday party was happening a few lanes over ... Where often running took me through parts of the city that were previously unencountered blank canvases, today I was running through a part of town that was saturated in memories.

The Running Factory, where my group running experience started, is on Wyandotte Street East, and as I ran by, two employees who were standing in the parking lot shouted encouragement to me. They had both run the Detroit earlier that day, and I could see their medals around their necks. I thought about stopping to chat, but I didn't want to throw off my run and sabotage my chance to gain the running-shaped hole.

Besides, if I stopped, I would be tempted to go inside the shop and peruse the racks for new running shirts and shorts. Running and weight loss had awakened the clothes shopper in me. I was able to walk into popular, trendy clothing stores and buy pants and shirts straight off the rack instead of searching desperately in the big-and-tall shops for something that fit and didn't look like it was designed for a septuagenarian. Over the previous few months, my dimensions had changed dramatically, and clothes ceased to chafe. This allowed me to expand my wardrobe into areas of fashion — current, youthful, complimentary to the body — that I had not been able to access in the plus-size market, where I had spent most of my adult life.

People were saying nice things about how I looked. In July 2013, my former newspaper colleague and LTR Clinic leader Kelly Steele had written an article for the *Windsor Star* about my transformation through running. This was responsible, in part, for the phone call from Shiva that had set all of this in motion.

Little River Bridge, located where Wyandotte Street crosses the Little River, is not much more than a sidewalk on a traffic access ramp spanning a local canal that's about twenty metres wide. I charged over that bridge like a man possessed. I had trained like a maniac and downed a lot of White Wasp heading into that fall. At the bridge's crown, I was about 7.5 kilometres into the run, and it was at that point that I knew what I was going to do. It was never my clear-cut, stated intention to run 21.1 kilometres that day. My Facebook post really only promised a "long run," leaving the door open to a half-marathon distance to mirror that morning's road races in Detroit. But now I knew that that was my goal. I felt that good.

Once on the other side of the bridge, I took a hard right-hand turn down onto the Ganatchio Trail where it winds through the woods known as Riverside Kiwanis Park. Following the trail south, I arrived at McHugh Street, and then I took a lap around a storm retention reservoir called Aspen Lake before looping back into the woods for the return trip to where the trail spills out onto its trunk line at Riverside Drive.

I'd managed to occupy the running-shaped hole pretty successfully over the first half of the run, but I'd sucked down all the Gu gels I'd socked away in the small pocket of my hydration belt and drained all the White Wasp from the bottle. My mindless focus was beginning to dissipate. But I wasn't ruminating on the things runners typically think about while they are running: pain, fatigue, thirst, hunger, home, bed, work, pressing family business, trivial household chores ... My thoughts were homing in on plain old boredom, and boredom's creeping terminal state: loneliness. In the end, running or not, it's always the loneliness. I wasn't worried about work, nor was I worried about chafing, even though it felt as if my left nipple was going to tear through the sweat-wicking fibre of my shirt. I wasn't worried about writing; I wasn't worried about money, aging, my health, my dad, my freedom, terrorism, the pets ... I wasn't worried about anything. I was deep into a one-man half-marathon, and I was just plain old sad and lonely and missing my wife and kids.

○ ○ ○

There's a playground incorporated into the trail system directly across Riverside Drive from the long-derelict Riverside Brewery. As I approached the playground, I spotted a familiar black Dodge Caravan in the parking lot. But it was empty. I slowed and stood there in the tree shade that canopied the playground. And then from behind various garbage cans, benches, and shrubs, I heard poorly stifled laughter. My children leapt out from their hiding places, nearly pulling me to the ground.

Of course, I'd been expecting them. I'd been carrying my phone in my hand the entire run to pre-arrange the playground meet-up for refuelling and a break. But in between my call and actually seeing Jennifer and the kids, I'd hit that wall of loneliness. Even though I knew I would see them at the rendezvous point, I had felt worried, as if I would not. I had felt that somehow it just wasn't going to work out, and I would be on my own until the end. Jennifer was there bearing bottles of cold White Wasp — one that I could drink from directly and one to replenish the bottle on my hydration belt — and plastic containers of frozen berries, pineapple, and melon. I was 12.5 kilometres into the run.

I stayed with them there in the parking lot for about three minutes, recharging the psychic batteries.

"Aren't you guys super proud of your dad?!"

There were lots of huzzahs and agreement.

"Okay, next meet me at —"

"You're not done? How far are you running?"

"I'm running a half-marathon. I've got about eight-and-a-half kilometres to go."

I can't blame Jennifer for thinking I was done and inviting me to hop into the passenger seat. I must've looked a mess. I'd been running for nearly two hours, but I was not getting in the vehicle. There were 8.5 kilometres to go, and I knew I had something in the tank — something unspent: the guts that until very recently I had not been aware I possessed.

When she realized I was continuing, Jennifer said she was proud of me. People will often say they are proud of you right before you go off half-cocked and do something fully cocked. Those people, in my experience, have never themselves been cocked to any degree. They have no idea what they are encouraging you to do. They are just loving encouragers. My wife, Jennifer, bless her heart, is one of those people. But runners, I've learned, are all pretty much unstable. (Hence the running.) Just as you wouldn't take spiritual advice from an atheist, you should never take advice about running from a non-runner. Jennifer tries, and I think honestly does want to run. But, like me before I discovered the running-shaped hole,

Jennifer hasn't yet discovered that running is an answer to a lot of things, like craziness.

Not for the first time, I felt a deep pang of guilt for her not continuing with her own running (though years later she would tell me it was a dislike of the group running dynamic that drove her from the LTR Clinic).

We went over the rest of my route, and after a quick round of hugs and kisses, I was back on the path, westward on Riverside Drive. My loneliness — my homesickness — at least for now, was cured.

o   o   o

My pace was slowing; my form was starting to dissolve. But there was no quit in me. For once, I was not letting pain, fatigue, fear, and boredom rule my thoughts. When I dialed my phone mid-stride around the 19-kilometre mark, it wasn't to call in the rescue wagon, it was to tell Jennifer and the kids where to meet me. Thinking of the stretch of Riverside Drive ahead of me, I tried to estimate where they should park to watch me hit the 21.1 kilometres. Not just because I didn't want to have to walk around looking for them, or pass out in a pile of freshly raked leaves on someone's lawn waiting for them to track me down, but because I wanted them to be there at the finish line. It took a couple of hasty phone calls, calibrating and recalibrating the anticipated vicinity of the finish line, but in the end, I pretty much nailed it.

Just before the deconsecrated monolith of the former Our Lady of the Rosary Church at the corner of Riverside Drive and Drouillard Road, I turned down a vestigial spur of Cadillac Street that runs between the church and the Ford Motor Company power plant and there sat the black Caravan. I could hear Jennifer and the kids yelling and clapping. I looked down at my watch and ran about 30 metres past the minivan and stopped the GPS recording. It wasn't official, but I'd just run my first half-marathon — a total of 21.1 kilometres, at an average pace of 8:03 per kilometre, for a total time of 2:50:10.

It had not been a shitshow. If you run a half-marathon on a whim, and, upon completion, walk under your own power into your home and can happily make yourself a toasted tomato sandwich between soleus muscle and IT-band stretches, then you have not participated in a shitshow. Hubris, though? Any time you run a great distance on a whim, you are doing something inspired by something dangerously close to hubris. But when the foolish and tragic thing, the bittersweet and quixotic fall from romantic heights doesn't come, your achievements will no longer be seen as the product of overconfidence; they are more likely to be viewed as the result of good planning and preparation.

James hit me up in a Facebook chat session a few weeks later. We often shared book recommendations between Windsor and Ottawa. I had made sure to mention what a boon to my running his championing of walk breaks had been, and I told him about Team Koushik's strange demise.

"Well, the good news is you trained, and you were prepared to run your leg of the relay," James said. "That training won't be wasted."

"Oh, I ran," I said. "More than my leg."

When I had finished outlining my lonely, solitary feat to him, James said, "Man, that's even better than the Free Press. You ran the Me Press!"

o   o   o

When the Koushiks' Diwali party rolled around a couple of weeks later, Jennifer and I were on the guest list and attended at Shiva and Aruna's home in LaSalle. Shiva and I shared a laugh over his thinking he had registered the relay team, and I told him about the Me Press. There were no hard feelings. Diwali, after all, is the time for celebrating the triumph of good over evil. I celebrated, lean and mean, in a spanking new, perfectly proportioned, custom-tailored champagne-coloured kurta.

CHAPTER NINE

THE FOREST OF PATERNAL DISMAY: A NIGHT IN THE BLACK OAK

NOT TO OVERSTATE anything or be too dramatic, but on a cold winter's night just before Christmas 2013, a plot of ancient forest on the outskirts of town almost became my Gethsemane.

I was running several times per week, racking up over 100 kilometres per month; I'd even run a half-marathon and been greeted at its makeshift finish line by my cheering family. I'd lost over one hundred pounds, I was buying and wearing clothes I had never in my most sartorial fantasies imagined I was built for … and it had only been a year. A year since I could barely bring myself to walk around a neighbourhood park.

This kind of hindsight can work two ways: it can give you some perspective on how far you've come in a relatively short period of time, or it can give you *way too much* perspective on how far you've come in a relatively short period of time. Yes, losing over one hundred pounds and putting myself through the pains of distance running was incredibly difficult. But considering the rewards (physical, mental, emotional, and spiritual) and what was at stake (my life and the stability and well-being of my young family), it was hard to understand why I hadn't done any of this earlier.

I knew from lessons I'd learned in sobriety that it happened when it happened for a reason, and on the deepest spiritual level, I believe that to be true. But on the pragmatic, work-a-day level we all seem to be conditioned to foreground, I couldn't help but feel some residual guilt. What role did my alcoholism, my overeating, my obesity, and now, maybe, even the rigorous schedule of my running play in any of the emotional and developmental difficulties our children were experiencing as they grew up?

Were these conditions the fallout of my past behaviours? Had I bent the path before them and warped their worldviews before they had even opened their eyes and drawn their first breaths?

Nathanael's dysthymia, for example: a low-grade depression that just simmered away in the back of his psyche at all times, making him feel misunderstood, less-than, and lonely; given to bouts of weepiness and severe self-criticism, foul temper and overeating ... How could I not see my own genetic code writ large across all of this? Of the three, Nathanael bears the strongest resemblance to me. It wasn't a stretch to see him, nearly identical to me in stature and mood, following, almost unwittingly, in my toxic footsteps. What young man, wracked with feelings of worthlessness and self-consciousness, wants their morbidly obese father at their side, bursting out of his ill-fitting wardrobe, gasping for breath mid-sentence, the obvious and too-easy target of every cruel joke? It would get to a point where he would realize two things worked to relieve the pain: food, which he had already discovered, and alcohol, which I dreaded his ever taking even a passing liking to.

The doctors said Jonah was the typical middle child: slow to speak, floating below the social radar, picky about the food he put in his mouth. But Jonah took his dietary proclivities to an extreme level, subsisting largely on baloney, white rolls, Honey Nut Cheerios, No-Name brand chicken nuggets, and Nutella well into his teens. He loved watching cooking shows on television and was eager to help in the kitchen but wouldn't dare touch the mushroom omelette or Sunday roast he helped prepare. We asked him *why* he didn't eat things like fresh, non-processed meats, eggs, cheese, anything with gravy or sauce … any of the myriad things he would not touch. He had no answer. Either he truly could not communicate it, or he was unwilling to say that he limited his palate in order to maintain his natural leanness and athleticism at all costs, aware that if he broadened his gastronomic horizons, he was opening the floodgates to broadening his waistband toward obesity. He saw his father's glaring weakness and knew — instinctually, in his own quiet fashion — that his infuriatingly picky eating was his best defence against coming to resemble me in any physical way.

Where Nathanael's dysthymia predisposed him to brooding and self-searching, Thomasin's anxiety, though obviously rooted in her own existential stuff, was always externally focused: Would I, her father, die in my sleep? What if I had a heart attack at work? What if her brothers got sick and died? Who would take care of her and her brothers if Jen and I were in an accident? Were the doors locked, were the phones charged, was the stove turned off, was there enough gas in the van? Did we have enough money to pay for her field trip to the symphony? Did we have enough money to make it through Christmas?

Many children, once they apprehend that first spectre of mortality, whether it's through the death of a beloved pet or an elderly relative, will have these thoughts. But rather than fading over time, Thomasin's thoughts increased in frequency and escalated in severity until she was unable to sleep; until she was going through a litany of safety checks any time either Jen or I left the house. Odd, I often thought, how she was as free and psychically unencumbered as you could hope a child would be when it came to her own safety; that it was the adults she mainly worried about. I couldn't help but wonder if having an obese father, even if my obesity wasn't the root cause of her worry, exacerbated every single worry. I wondered if she was so anxious because she sensed my vulnerability and help-lessness, my own fear of being unable to help my family — to run to their aid, to swim them to shore, to carry them from a tragedy, to defend them from a deranged man in the streets — if, God forbid, there was ever a need.

Here was guilt. Here was the darkness I truly ran in. The dark-ness my children faced, the darkness Jennifer shouldered and nur-tured us through, putting her own emotional and mental health at risk.

o   o   o

Although I no longer felt the need to hide under cover of dark-ness when I ran, my meteoric ascent was not without its cautionary contrails.

About eight months after the Spring Thaw, on a sub-zero December night, I left the warm confines of our family home on Moy Avenue, dressed in my cold-weather running gear, and drove out to the desolate southwest corner of Windsor to a patch of an-cient old-growth forest on the banks of the Detroit River known as Black Oak Heritage Park. I'd gone from nearly housebound, imprisoned by self-consciousness and fear because of my weight, to someone who went out in the dead of night in the dead of winter to test his physical limits. Trail running was good for that. Trail running in a polar vortex was even better.

The small gravel lot at the entrance to the park was deserted when I pulled in. Stepping out into the night air, I felt the cold immediately penetrating the thin layers of my running tights and jacket. I donned my running gloves and toque and, fussing to fit my phone into one of my jacket's small pockets, opted to leave it in the van and run without my running app tracking my progress. The running magazines and gurus often touted the occasional technology-free run.

I knew it would take me just over an hour to travel the roughly 10 kilometres of looping trails that are packed into the Black Oak's one hundred hectares before emerging from the trees into the safe confines of the parking lot. The best way to activate the moisture-wicking and heat-retaining tech fibres of my winter gear was to get moving, so I shut the van door, zipped up my jacket, pulled my Merino-wool Buff up over the lower half of my face, and set out on this solitary race against myself — my weight, my appetites, my nature, my fears.

A wood-chip path led through an open savannah into the forest proper, and once you were in amongst the old-growth forest, the trails narrowed to the width of footfalls and began to loop deviously around the densely packed trees. It was one of those nights when the air is so cold and still that you can hear the crystalline tinkling of the snow. I turned on my headlamp, which illuminated an orb about 10 metres in front of me, but in the winding dark of Black Oak, I had little choice but to keep my gaze locked on the trail, a black ribbon of compacted earth that ran through the snow-white woods, just a metre or so in front of me. Soon, the clicking of the snow and the snapping of the branches disappeared from my consciousness, and all I could hear was my breath and my footfalls.

The trail emerges from the forest at one point and crosses a second savannah, behind the towering silos of the Dainty Rice plant. At another point, it drops down into a dry gulch that, when it's possible to get surer footing, you can clear with a single leap. The wild, natural world of the wood is divided by a rail line, which passes through the park, bisecting it from east to west, and terminates at the towering grain elevators and derricks of the Morton Terminal at the river's edge, just beyond the Black Oak's southern reach.

Although this was my first time running in Black Oak at night, it was maybe my tenth time there in the past two months, so I was familiar with the trail. I hit all the now-familiar landmarks and vistas at all the expected intervals.

Running in Black Oak offers definite physical benefits: varied cardio conditioning resulting from the wide variety of terrain encountered and the building of stabilizing muscles in the feet and ankles as a result of the frequent tight turns. Running there also brought me a lot of peace. The trunks of trees constantly passing in the periphery providing a trance-like visual stimulus that made the time spent winding through the hardwood, pushing myself toward exhaustion, slip by. And the truly great thing about running in Black Oak was that as long as you stay on the trail — *if you commit to the path* — it *always* loops back around to the parking lot. You don't really have to worry about where exactly you are. If you trust in the path, it will lead you home.

And then I ran full tilt into a deer. Sensing its presence at the last second, I looked up into the headlamp-illuminated trail in front of me and saw it standing there: a large buck with a menacing rack. It was too late to stop. I let out a heaving grunt as I collided with its flank and hindquarters. It barely moved. We stood inches apart, staring at each other in the cold, grey light of the lamp, our breath intermingling in the beam. He held his taut pose on the trail, seemingly still convinced I could not see him despite our recent collision. He scraped a black slash in the trail with a hoof, snorted once, and went arcing off through the frosty foliage. There was a snapping of branches and the briefest rustling of brittle leaves, and then all was quiet again.

I looked down at my body; the lamplight revealed a fine coating of deer hair glinting on my black running tights — fawn against the neon green and royal blue of my running jacket. It was hard to say how long I stood there, more enchanted than startled from my run-in with the deer, but it was probably less than thirty seconds. I knew I was about forty minutes and roughly 6.5 kilometres into my run — about twenty-five minutes out from the van. The temperature was dropping — it was supposed to hit minus twenty degrees Celsius that night. It was time to get moving.

As I continued along the trail, I kept my head up and stayed more aware of my surroundings, knowing that in those tight confines a second encounter with the buck — or possibly a whole herd of deer, simply looking for a warm spot to huddle together for the night — wasn't out of the question.

A downed tree crossed the path. I hurdled it without incident and was in the middle of thinking, *That wasn't here last time I —*

For the second time that night, I stopped dead in my tracks. I was staring at a chain-link fence, which in and of itself was nothing out of the ordinary … except it wasn't supposed to be there, not in this part of the Black Oak, not in any part of the Black Oak I had ever encountered. The trail simply entered a banked curve and button-hooked back into the trees, away from the fence, which stretched in both directions as far as my headlamp would allow me to see. It was what rose in the distance, beyond the cruel twists of wire that lined the top of the fence, that sent a bolt of cold dread and disbelief through my steaming body: Morton Terminal, with its winking lights that speckled the towering grain elevators in a bokeh-dot array. I heard the ambient mechanical whine of various cranes and conveyors, saw the giant lake freighters at rest along the quay, so close I could see Christmas lights strung in the windows along their bridges.

I was a long way from where I was supposed to be. Instead of being a matter of minutes from the parking lot, I was now at the farthest possible southwestern corner of the park, somewhere I had never been. I didn't even know the trail came back this way. Now, an hour into the run, I was thirsty, hungry, tired, and, most distressingly, cold. And the temperature was still dropping.

I turned to survey the forest behind me. The dark, thin band of the trail snaked off into sfumato of snow and trees. It coiled everywhere: distinct loops that at times nearly touched, like oil bubbles in water, separated by the merest rind of snow. But where moments before the unwavering and true nature of the path had been its great, peace-bringing strength, the fact that the loops came so close to touching without ever actually doing so, was now its most maddening feature.

Colliding with the deer, I realized, may have resulted in me inadvertently stepping onto an adjacent loop of trail, virtually indistinguishable even in broad daylight, from the loop of the trail I had been on just prior to impact. Then, when I had continued on my way, I was inadvertently heading into unfamiliar territory, travelling deeper into the woods than I had ever ventured before.

How much time passed between the collision with the buck and hurdling the log? I wondered. It seemed like it had been just a few minutes, but the only reference point I had was the trance-like repetition of running through trees on a winding meditative path. My body was telling me I had run what felt like 3 or 4 kilometres, which is why I thought I was coming to the end of the trail. Yet, here I was, off in some Black Oak backwater, at least a kilometre as the crow flies beyond what I had previously thought was the southern extremity of the trail. Adding up all the twisting and turning made the 3 or 4 kilometres I felt I had travelled make sense ... but it was all speculation.

The timelines and distances were all out of sync. Everything was distorted. Maybe this was the early cognitive dissolution symptomatic of hypothermia? Of course, in all this consulting of the trail and trying to figure out how far I had travelled, I had become disoriented, unable to determine which direction I had been travelling. I couldn't even determine where the log I had hurdled was located. It should have been somewhere in my field of vision because surely only seconds had passed between encountering it and arriving at the fence ... But I couldn't even accurately determine how much time had passed between the buck and the log. It's unlikely my sense of time had become more accurate the more lost I became. So, which strand of the path had I arrived from? Inspecting the ground at my feet, I could see from the mess of footprints around me that I had now crossed back and forth from one loop of trail to another more than once in my quandary.

As panic rose in my chest and the temperature continued to plummet, I tried to come to terms with the long run that was ahead of me if I wanted to get back to the van. Should I head back the way I had come (if I actually knew which direction that was) knowing that *that* was an hour's run, or should I continue the way I'd been going? Was that less than an hour back to the parking lot? Did it even lead there at all? What if I just left the section of the trail I was standing on and stepped over onto the loop that passed a few feet to my right? Would I be slashing twenty-five minutes off my efforts to get back to the warmth and safety of the van, or would I be tacking on a heedless slog into the winter dawn, in what I was beginning to think of as my desperate pursuit of survival?

I don't remember what caused me to make the decision I made, but I found myself running again in what I figured was the direction I had been travelling when I was stopped by the fence. My hands ached from the cold seeping into my running gloves. Beneath my Buff, partially frozen from my exhalations, my nose and cheeks burned. My toes could have been missing inside my shoes for all I could feel of them. Added to this, the guiding light of my headlamp was starting to flicker, its candlepower fading as the cold sapped the batteries, and my decision to go tech-free on this run was starting to look like the kind of tragic final decision people whisper about in small groups at funerals.

Except it wasn't me I was worried about. My worry was focused on Jennifer and the kids, who would doubtless be worried sick about my having left the house for a run after supper and not returning. My thoughts raced beyond my control, and soon I was envisioning a police cruiser gliding to a halt in front of the house, two constables approaching the door, caps in hand, Jennifer collapsing to her knees in the exact spot I had been kneeling to retrieve that Luke Skywalker figure from under the piano when I learned my mother was dead, the children gradually catching on that their father was gone — perished in a woodlot; found frozen in a deer-abandoned hollow; a victim of exposure, but apparently also having been kicked and gored to death by an aggressive buck.

This was the never-ending sadness I had inflicted on them through my hubris, the enduring, life-long absence of their husband and father, right when he was finally getting his eating and weight under control. I had ruined their lives. My selfish, adventure-seeking behaviour, this new-found obsession with running, had led me back into the centre of their lives and then straight out again, petering out after ricochetting around like an entropic bullet in one of the country's most historically and ecologically significant stands of oak. I had failed them. Again.

I had strayed from the path. Inadvertently or no, it spelled certain doom.

More than once, I stopped, listening for traffic, the conveyors of the terminal, the baying of hounds, and the call of my rescuers, summoned by my frantic wife, desperate for my safe return. I have no idea how long I ran. Hours had passed, surely. My spatial and directional sense were confounded by the Black Oak. The phone I had opted to leave in the van rather than fuss with had a GPS compass, mapping apps, and a flashlight. It was also, obviously, a *telephone*, which I could have used to call for help. I could have called home to say good-bye.

If I live, I will never leave my phone behind again, I promised myself. *If I live, I will make my family proud of me. I will make them proud of my running. I will write a book about it.*

I just kept running. I just went around and around in the Black Oak, tears frozen in my eyelashes, resisting the urge to change my loop, to try my hand with a new timeline. I just kept running. And then I felt gravel beneath my foot. The path widened to a two-lane cart path and eventually let out onto the frosted savannah, then the parking lot.

The van sat stolidly in the night. With frantic, frozen hands, I fished the fob out of the small pocket inside the waistband of my running tights. Once inside, I started the engine, cranked the heat, and sat there whimpering as the engine's output gradually warmed me. When I could feel my hands, I fished the phone out of the console and hit Jennifer's number on speed dial.

"Hi!" she said, in the same excited tone of voice she would have used had I been calling from my desk at the newspaper.

"Oh my God," I heaved. "I'm so sorry. I got lost, I hit a deer —"

"You hit a deer with the van?" Now she was worried.

"No, no, I ran into a deer — we hit each other on the trail, and I got lost and I left my phone in the van because I thought I knew where I was going and … I just didn't know if I was going to make it."

"Oh, honey — are you okay? You sound upset. Are you in the van now — hold on a sec — Nathanael, can you help your brother with that? I don't want it to get broken … Okay, sorry. They are being monkeys. But you're okay? You're on your way home?"

I could hear the kids playing and laughing in the background. I could hear the TV. "Yeah, I'm — wait, what time is it?" I asked, looking at the time on the van stereo at the same time Jennifer told me it was about twenty after seven. In the evening.

Not one thirty in the morning. Not just before dawn the next day. It was 7:20 in the evening of the same day that I had left the house for my run. The kids weren't even in bed yet. I'd only been gone for a little over two hours. My supper, I was told, was keeping warm in the oven for me.

I drove home. I even stopped and picked up two coffees and a box of doughnut holes for the kids. I figured I'd run at least 20 kilometres that night. For all I knew, it was my longest run to date. I'd gone from being a man on the very precipice of losing his family to a man who had made a decision to make good on a promise to his mother and run *toward* that family; to run toward health, longevity, and a greater sobriety than the one I had been living with since the days of my last drink. I'd made a decision to once again change my life, and my life did indeed change. I had not failed them. I had stayed on the path after all.

CHAPTER TEN

YOU'RE GOING TO NEED MORE STORMS

WHEN YOU ARE in pain, you will do almost anything to relieve the pain. You may abandon your composure, compromise your values — in other words, do things you would not under normal circumstances do in order to feel better, even temporarily. Which is how I came to be lying on a small plot of grass with my legs in the air, crying out for mercy, a man perched on top of me, shouting instructions while he pressed the heel of his hand into my buttocks and rearranged my limbs.

All in plain sight of the cyclists, dog walkers, and parents with their children at the playground metres away.

Lots of good stories start with a dare, and this story — full of improbability, tough luck, heartbreak, and actual physical pain — is no different. On New Year's Day, 2014, Kira texted me from Toronto and challenged me to join her in running the Detroit Free

Press Marathon. It was ten months away. I was registered by lunchtime. The two members of our nameless running entity were united in our commitment to log the lonely distances, separated by hundreds of kilometres, and meet in the start corrals come that October dawn in downtown Detroit.

The next several months were devoted to maintaining my running schedule through the winter and preparing for the arduous marathon training season, which was set to begin in June. I ran my second Spring Thaw 5K, besting my time from the previous year by more than twelve minutes. In May I ran my first "official" half-marathon, Windsor's Le Chocolat, in 2:42:45 — besting my "unofficial" Me Press time by over seven minutes on a looping, mind-numbingly repetitive tour of the Windsor waterfront that, although it measured 21.1 kilometres, left me feeling as if I had been cheated out of a real half-marathon experience. Had it been a looping, riverfront course in St. Louis, London, or even on the Detroit side of the Detroit River, I probably would have felt a lot different about Le Chocolat. But seeing as how I rely so much on the visual stimulus of an ever-changing cityscape to ward off boredom, treading over the same territory four times in the same long-distance race was pretty uninspiring and demoralizing.

I turned forty about six weeks later. I weighed 228 pounds — 140 pounds down from where I started eighteen months earlier when I set a goal of losing one hundred pounds by my fortieth birthday. To mark the occasion, I woke up early and ran a half-marathon — 21.1 kilometres that took me deep into the west side of the city before circling back to home along the waterfront. I was four minutes slower than my Le Chocolat time, but the fact that there was a time when, at thirty years old (a year sober but nearly immobile and in constant pain and discomfort from pushing four hundred pounds), I was closer to death than I was on my fortieth birthday made any discussion of pace and time absolutely irrelevant. I felt deeply satisfied and virile.

Other major life changes were afoot: after a decade, the sheen had definitely worn off being a one-man newsroom at a weekly newspaper, and at Jennifer's insistence, I'd resigned from my position as the editor, senior reporter, reviewer, and photographer at the *LaSalle Post*. She knew I was miserable working for a newspaper under Postmedia's "digital first" death march toward the end of print journalism. I was burned out from the weekly race against the clock that took place in annular loops within the ceaseless, seasonal news cycle of the small-town newspaper. The stress was bad, the money was worse, and when Jennifer pitched me on the idea of simply staying at home and writing full-time, I didn't hesitate to give my two-weeks notice.

Writing news copy all day was no substitute for working on poetry and fiction, and the sense of detachment I felt from my work only added to my waning enthusiasm for print journalism. Running, of course, helped with the stress load, but an aggressive, ambitious marathon training schedule meant any writing projects had lapsed into a state of near dormancy. The novel, which was older than our oldest child, had been in a state of protracted hibernation for several years. Poetry, which, for me, always just kind of happens when it happens, hadn't really been happening since the publication of *Campfire Radio Rhapsody* three years earlier. Whether I ran before going to work in the morning, or after work in the evening, at the end of the day I had nothing left to give to my creative pursuits, and so I spent what little time remained each day trying to be an active and present husband and father.

But with the 42.2 kilometres of the Detroit Marathon drawing closer, all of my writing was on the backburner. I was wholly focused on running. Jennifer said nothing. She knew where I was (out in the city somewhere), and she knew what I was doing (changing my life). I barely remember any of that summer. It seems I was either out running, or I was eating or sleeping. On the nights I would try to stay up and write, I would wake up at my desk, stiff and awash in drool.

Kira and I would check in via text message every few days, updating each other on run duration, training schedule, stress, and general exhaustion levels. Many more experienced runners complimented me on my enthusiasm, but they also cautioned me against running my first full marathon too soon. Overtraining, they said, was the quickest route to an injury. I would smile and nod; I had decided, however, that their advice did not pertain to me. The more I ran, the more I occupied the running-shaped hole; the more I occupied the running-shaped hole, the more I could reside outside of the stress of training for a full marathon. I could focus on increasing my pace, the resulting Personal Bests in my 5K and 10K times that I was achieving nearly every time I stepped out in my running gear, and my decreasing weight.

Then, about ten weeks out from the Detroit Marathon, my phone blew up with a series of text messages from Kira. The person who had challenged me to join her in the Detroit Marathon was out of the race as the result of a non-running-related injury. Doctor's orders.

It takes a strong runner to admit to any kind of injury. It also takes a strong runner to show up in the start corrals for his first marathon without the person he saw himself struggling along with between kilometre 22 and 42.2. I was going to be the lone ice-cream cone standard bearer heading into Detroit.

The best way to combat the fear of underperforming and dropping out of my first full marathon, I figured, was to get super-uncomfortable and join the Running Factory's Marathon and Half-Marathon Clinic. My inclinations for solitude were not going to do me any favours. My game plan going into the clinic was to generally keep to myself and somehow withstand the twin pressures of running my first full marathon and being the last person standing in what, in hindsight, was maybe a ludicrous challenge to have accepted. I was stressed out. And I was frightened. All that meant, though, was that I needed to train longer and harder. The fortunes of our entire two-person running group rested squarely and solely on me.

○ ○ ○

The good folks at the Running Factory must see guys like me coming from several kilometres away: galvanized by our new-found running successes; blinded by our too-close-to-the-sun penchant for hubris; numbed by overzealousness to the rough reality that diminished returns lie ahead; and all but bound to overtrain. Indeed, my copy of the training manual we were all given as part of the Running Factory's Marathon and Half Marathon Training Clinic has more than a few passages marked for future reference, including a cautionary note in the "Training Roadblocks" section that warns about overtraining and cutting yourself some slack if you missed a training run. I dutifully underlined this road-tested advice in blue ink and then promptly forgot it.

I don't want to use age or a lack of running experience as an excuse. And I don't want to use my being what is typically, though non-specifically, classified as a "bigger runner," as an excuse — it is true, though, that being anything above 180 pounds is considered by some to be beyond the physiognomic pale. The only excuse I have is that I lack perspective. I simply don't see things correctly, and as I have learned in my recovery from alcoholism, I am frequently wrong. My disease is one of perception. Whether it was alcohol or food, I only ever saw the maximum.

With booze, I had adopted the old "one's too many, a thousand isn't enough" mentality. If you offered me a beer and opened your fridge to reveal the five beers you currently had in your possession,

Robert Earl Stewart

I would refuse your offer because unless you could assure me someone was showing up with a full case, or there were plans to vacate your woefully understocked abode for the lush pastures of the neighbourhood hotel or the glittering nightmare of downtown, there was no use in even getting started. Nothing was worse than draining two beers and fighting off sleep while being driven mad by an unslakable desire. Of course, aside from the continuous quantity-based calculation and fretting of the alcoholic, my diseased perceptions were based more in the ego — my entire personality was consumed by how people saw me, my flaws, my imperfections. And, as messed up as it may sound, during the fifteen years of my active drinking, I wanted people to see me as a heavy drinker.

But with food, it was a bit different. The same diseased perception was at work, but I preferred it if people didn't see me. I was so ashamed of myself at every stop along the scale, from 260, to 300, to 350 pounds and beyond, that eating, even after a decade of sobriety, was the only thing that could make me feel better about myself. My gluttony allowed me to focus, however dubiously and briefly, on something other than how uncomfortable and embarrassed I always felt.

So, in becoming a runner, I was all but predestined to overdo it. Once I started stepping into and filling up that running-shaped hole and feeling (and watching) my life change, my distorted perception was going to outpace the limits of my physiognomy. All the cautionary paragraphs ever written in all the running manuals would not have been able to convince me to do things like fit a marathon training schedule into my life, rather than fit what remained of my life into my marathon training schedule; understand that the schedule I was given was a suggestion and not a mandate. When I looked at the Running Factory's marathon training schedule, I failed to see that on any given day of training, there were three options listed, three distances that you could choose to run that

168

day, given your experience level and how you were feeling overall. I always chose the longest distance because that was the one my ego locked on.

On the first night of group training, there was not much difference in the three distances, with Level 1 running 5K, Level 2 running 6.5K, and Level 3 running 8K. Of course, I ran the 8K at a pace of 7:09/kilometre for a 51:19 total time, doing so in a humidity that sapped my energy and left me feeling disappointed in my performance. A month into the clinic, the gap between Level 1 and Level 3 was widening. On the first Saturday of August, for example, Level 1 runners had 11K for their long run. Level 3 was slated for 14.5K. A 3.5-kilometre difference. Both distances were more than achievable; both would have been perfectly decent runs, and depending on how hard I wanted to push myself (ever conscious of running slightly below my expected race pace for the 42.2K in Detroit), the run could have been relaxed, or challenging.

Well, I ran 16.12K because — even though there is that line in the clinic manual that says, "If you miss a training session here or there, [it] will not make or break your race" — two nights before I had to cut a run short for the perfectly reasonable fact that I had to get to Jonah's baseball practice, and only ran 8.3K of what was supposed to be a 9.5K — the maximum posted training distance for that day, of course. I was consumed by the need to make up that 2.2K shortcoming. If you do the math, you'll see that I fell 580 metres short of making it up.

The game in my head — the head ruled by my diseased perception — was on. And even in trying to excel, I was already falling short, which only made me try to tack on a few more kilometres next time. The times that I would tack on the extra distance and feel particularly pleased (and possibly exhausted) would soon be overshadowed by a run that fell short. On the rare occasion that I would allow myself to consider running the lesser distance, the

17.5K instead of the 19K, a familiar and diseased thought process would take over: *Why run 17.5K when 19K would be better?* It's no different than, *Why get the single-pound burger when the two-pound burger would clearly be better?* And in the end, it starts to resemble — and this scares the shit out of me — my relationship with alcohol: one's too many, a thousand's not enough. Whether you're talking kilometres or drinks, the end result is sickness and pain.

And the pain did come. You can deny it for a long time — days, weeks, maybe even months — but eventually that day comes when the pain paralyzes the stubborn, denial-addled liar inside of you long enough for reality to slip through the chinks in the stupid fucking armour of pride you've been running around town in, thinking you're really winning this battle against the rigours of marathon training ... And you realize you're injured.

For weeks I'd been running as if everything — my fortunes, Kira's recovery, the way I felt about myself, and, most importantly, the way my wife and children and friends and colleagues thought of me — resided in my performance in the Detroit Free Press Marathon. The weight of all of this rested across my shoulders like a blood-soaked rood. As it turned out, everything rested on my hips.

My left hip was a mess. The result, quite simply, of marathon training: the big ramp up in mileage and hours spent pounding the pavement. I'd gone from running three half-marathons over a seven-month span, to running that distance (21.1 kilometres) every weekend through July and into August. The importance of striking a balance between being undertrained and healthy and being overtrained and injured was something I had been doling out as sage advice to other runners, but I had failed to put this piece of wisdom into practice in my own running game.

I kept training this way, my pace gradually diminishing below any kind of "slightly slower than race pace" threshold, my laboured stride becoming increasingly hard to ignore, until the night of

August 19, 2014, at the Marathon and Half-Marathon Clinic group run at Blue Heron Lake, the large, trail-entwined manmade hill on the Windsor-Tecumseh border. It had been a particularly stormy summer, and we'd been having a lot of violent weather on the nights of the clinic. There'd been more than a few nights when the clinic leaders cancelled the workout due to lightning, torrential rain, hail, and, the previous week, tornado warnings (two small, F1 tornadoes had touched down on the other side of town in South Windsor). But that night held no promise of rain. It was, in fact, blisteringly hot.

I didn't even make it through that evening's 2K warm-up around the water retention pond. Each step required a conscious heaving around of the leg, my foot landed devoid of any range of motion on the pavement, giving me no propulsion and completely throwing off my stride as my right leg came racing forward in a failed attempt to make it look like I was not limping, but instead making it look as if I had never run as much as a step in my life because of an extremely pronounced limp. I lagged far behind the rest of the group, and when the pain was too much to bear, I stopped running.

I limped all the way around to the foot of the Blue Heron hill, where the clinic participants were lining up to begin that night's battery of drills and hill repeats, to pick up my hydration belt, then I turned around and limped the 300 metres back to the lot where the van was parked. It was a long, painful, and humiliating retreat. No one else, to my knowledge, had ever walked away from a clinic session before. Everyone seemed limber and hale, their strides natural and easy, their stress levels low to non-existent. I could not look back at them. This was the runner's equivalent to a walk of shame. I wanted to get back to the van as quickly as my messed-up hip would allow, not just so I could ease myself into the driver's seat and maybe pass out from the pain, but maybe also have a good cry before doing so.

But as I crossed the street into the parking lot, Kyle, one of the clinic leaders, was just arriving at Blue Heron. He was a physiotherapy technician: the person who teaches you the stretches and strengthening exercises the physiotherapist recommends after manipulating and adjusting you. His face was full of empathy and concern as he approached. I was teary, in agony, and embarrassed. Within seconds, he had me lying in the cool grass that ringed the parking lot, which is how I came to be therapeutically adjusted in front of that evening's crowd of park-goers, who were being quickly disabused of their naïveté with regard to the running community.

It hurt like mad, and Kyle apologized as I winced and whimpered under his professional touch. He helped me to my feet and convinced me to jog slowly and lightly down the sidewalk with him so he could check some things with my form and gait. He could see just from our little run down the sidewalk that my lower back, where the multifidus muscle engages with and controls the glutes and the muscles, tendons, and fascia tissues of the hip girdle, was weak. The marathon training had not strengthened this area. In fact, running won't strengthen this area. But strengthening exercises will. All the marathon training had done was tear up and inflame the tissue around my hip and iliotibial (IT) band.

The pain on that night gave me a moment of clarity; I finally had the ability to honestly and realistically appraise the situation and act on what I saw. The pain was mental. It was emotional. It was in my head and heart. It stopped being about mileage and pace, and it suddenly was all about how great I felt when I was running. And when I was running in pain, it was just a misguided attempt to fill up that running-shaped hole.

The whole sorry scenario reminded me of that part in *Catch-22* when Yossarian and Doc Daneeka are discussing how pilots like Yossarian's friend, Orr, can be grounded and prevented from flying any more missions. Their discussion of the novel's central paradox, like almost every bit of dialogue in Joseph Heller's monumental novel about bomber pilots on the Mediterranean island of Pianosa during the Second World War, is absolutely brilliant and maddening. All of the bomber pilots on Pianosa, Doc explains to Yossarian, are certifiably crazy and, as such, cannot fly any more missions. But he cannot ground them until they ask to be grounded. However, as soon as they ask to be grounded, expressing rational concern for their own safety and well-being, they are deemed sane, and Doc can no longer ground them. I was in a similar situation: I needed running in my life because it was the thing that helped me work things out in my head; not being able to run made running become the thing in my head that needed to be worked out. So, I was willing to run and risk further injury, pain, and mental turmoil, just for a day or so of peace. Put another, more Heller-esque way:

> ... *a concern for one's own health and safety in the face of injuries that were real and immediate was the process of a rational mind. I was sane and needed to stop running. All I had to do was admit it; and as soon as I did and stopped running, I would be crazy and would have to run. I would be crazy to go on more runs, and sane if I didn't, but if I was crazy, I had to go running. If I ran, I was crazy and shouldn't run; but if I didn't run, I was crazy and had to.*

My peace of mind was shot, and I sensed the spectre of depression and its attendant paranoias and worries lurking just beneath the surface of everything I thought, said, or did. That was enough to get me to admit I needed help.

I went hobbling on what felt like stumps attached to suddenly palsied, geriatric hips, to Corey, a highly recommended physiotherapist.

After putting my hip through a battery of manipulations, noting the various grindings, hitches, and clickings from deep in my socket, Corey pulled up a stool and was quiet for a moment. "When is your run again?" she asked, "October what?"

"October nineteenth," I told her.

She looked over her shoulder at a calendar on the wall. "And you're doing the full?"

"The full, yes."

"How has training been going?" she asked. "Other than this."

I told Corey about the Marathon and Half-Marathon Clinic, that the training schedule was hard, that the person I had registered for Detroit with was injured and wasn't going to be able to run, that several of the clinic's group-training runs at the Blue Heron hill had been cut short or cancelled because of the menacing storms that swept through the region seemingly every Tuesday night that summer.

"Well, you're going to need more storms," Corey said.

She knew she was breaking my heart. And I was foolish enough, even with this pain, this enormous hitch in my stride, to think she was going to have good news for me. She said even with thrice-weekly clinic visits, she doubted I would be ready for Detroit — full or half. She was recommending a complete cessation of running, at least for a week to ten days — preferably two weeks, if I could stand it.

I considered my days going forward without running. That passage in the Marathon and Half-Marathon Clinic Training workbook — the one I had underlined in blue ink and promptly ignored — about not overtraining leapt to mind.

Doing all the physiotherapist-recommended exercises was one thing, but the most active role I was going to have to play in my own recovery involved exercising my patience. Patience and recovery had gone together in my life since April 11, 2003. Despite that, and although patience is always something I pray for and work on, it is not something I am especially good at.

I was coming to terms with the fact that running was not always going to be awesome and healthy and injury-free. But I had also gained insight into something else, something much more unsettling: I did not enjoy the time commitment and the stress of training for a marathon. The past eight months had been amongst the most stressful in my life. Where was the calming, freeing influence of running I had fallen in love with?

CHAPTER ELEVEN

FREE PRESS PRISONER

I GIVE PEOPLE who turn out to cheer on runners on race day a lot of credit. I appreciate them being out there when I run by, whether it's a 5K or a half-marathon. Even the well-wishers who say nice things as I run past them on the street or on a trail get my thanks and respect. Lacking this innate generosity myself, I am always touched when I encounter these people in the wild.

My friend Jeffery, who lives along Riverside Drive East, goes so far as to buy crates of oranges and, along with his wife, children, and his old Delta Chi fraternity brothers, makes a big annual thing out of slicing them up and handing fresh wedges to Free Press runners as they stream by his home, eastbound toward the Windsor-Detroit Tunnel during the international leg of the race. He displays such an incredible amount of *joie de vivre, ésprit de corps, je ne sais quoi*, and all the other French qualities I lack.

When the 37th Detroit Free Press Marathon start horn went off at 7:00 a.m. on October 19, 2014, I was in bed. Sleeping.

Jeffery and his team handed out two hundred pounds of sliced oranges. Photos of the aftermath — Riverside Drive littered with rinds of pith and peel smiling up from the gutter — were posted online. I missed all of this. I was in bed. Sleeping. When a bunch of my friends and running acquaintances made the turn off Goyeau Street into the Windsor-Detroit Tunnel for the return trip stateside, I remained abed, asleep. When the overall winner, twenty-seven-year-old Mike Andersen of Walled Lake, Michigan, crossed the finish line at 2:24:54, I hadn't even stirred. I think, subconsciously, I was trying to hide my shame by staying beneath the sheets until around 1:00 p.m., when, had I been running, I likely would have been finishing and surrendering my hips and multifidus muscles to the nearest race official or oblivious spectator, for proper disposal.

"Excuse me, ma'am. Will you throw this in the garbage for me?"
"Why, what is it?"
"It's just my ass, and some other shit."

Where had my passion for running — that throwing-caution-to-the-wind insouciance that a year before had seen me run my own 21.1K on the day of Detroit — disappeared to? This year, I slept in and had my laptop delivered to me in bed so I didn't have to do anything. Yes, I was injured, but to not even get out of bed and cheer on the people who had trained just as hard — and more successfully! — than me as they ran their guts out in a road race across parts of two countries? (There are probably many French words that could be used to describe my petulant malcontentedness.)

I spent a couple of hours lying there with my laptop, watching as my Facebook news feed filled up with photos from both sides of the border as able-bodied runners got out there and ran their race. Races are a huge, joyous business. Even small races in remote locales come to resemble festivals unfolding around a parade of sweaty, exhausted, and smiling people in tight, colourful clothes.

The Free Press is no small race, though. Some twenty-seven thousand people ran some aspect of the 37th running: whether the Full, the International Half, the U.S. Half, the Marathon Relay, or the 5K. For nearly all of it, I was hiding from the world, taking only the occasional peek at the race conditions, results, and finisher photos on my laptop.

Eventually, I got up and tried to pretend the race hadn't happened. Or, that if it had, it had nothing to do with me. In my mind, for that Sunday, I wanted to be a non-runner. With the laptop closed and my phone turned off, I wouldn't have to watch as everyone I knew finished their run. Already, I had seen the posted photos of people I knew, kicking toward the finish, holding up their medals, hugging loved ones while wrapped in thermal foil. My response to several of these photos: *He runs?! She finished her second full?! His time was what?!*

I was at once proud of their efforts and jealous of their success. And jealousy, like pride, also goeth before the fall.

Nathanael found me staring blankly into the refrigerator, confronted with naught but yogurt and romaine lettuce, when what I wanted to see was baked goods and ice cream. He asked me what was wrong — he had probably heard one of my deep, existential sighs. "You look sad," he said.

"I'm upset that I didn't run the Detroit Full this morning," I said.

"Because of your injury," he said emphatically, reminding me that it wasn't for lack of running."

I avoided his eyes. "Yes, because of that."

Jonah entered the kitchen. "Remember that time I helped you make all that food at Christmas and then I refused to eat any of it? Well, you said that it was okay because sometimes all the work is more important than what most people might think is the goal."

"That sounds like something I would say," I admitted.

"Well, you did all the work. You just couldn't do that part that most people think is the important part at the end."

"It's frustrating," I said. "It's more than that."

Jonah didn't have anything else to say, so he just wrapped his lanky arms around his brother and I and said, "Group hug."

Sunday errand-running provided ample distraction and ample excuse to not go for even the most cursory of runs. Of course, I was hyper-conscious of running into anyone I knew amongst the Sunday afternoon grocery-shopping crowd, envisioning conversations I didn't want to be a part of.

"Hey man, looking pretty good for a guy who ran the marathon this morning! No rest for the wicked, eh? What was your time?"

"Bob Stewart! I was thinking about you this morning when I saw all those pics from the Free Press Marathon in my news feed. How'd you make out? I know you were training like crazy. What was your time?"

None of that happened. I returned home within a few hours, laden with comfort food, but otherwise unaccosted. Of course, that all changed as soon as I fired up my phone to check for messages. A fresh barrage of soul-wrenching race stories awaited me in my Facebook, Twitter, Instagram, and Nike+ running feeds — stories that bore that wonderful stamp of improbability that running can make possible in your life but will sap your lifeforce if you're not running at the time. Stuff like: *The last time I saw her she was drunk and bumming a smoke off someone outside of a bar. That was in August. She must feel great having just completed her first half in one hour and thirty-three minutes!* and *Oh look, that guy who dropped out of the Marathon and Half-Marathon Clinic after two weeks because it was too hard and he didn't like being told he would probably need new shoes ran a 3:27 full marathon in basketball high-tops.*

If Sunday was a day for denial and judgment, Monday provided ample opportunity for second-guessing and guilty navel-gazing.

The plan was to get up, do some writing, all the while looking forward to that evening's run with the fall session of the Learn to Run Clinic at the Running Factory. First thing's first, though: I had to update my Facebook status. That simple and routine act ended up setting the tone for the entire day (and gave rise to this chapter). That status:

> The day after you *don't* run the Detroit Free Press Marathon is the perfect day to start turning all your notes on how angry and jealous you are into a chapter in your book about running the Detroit Free Press Marathon.

Things don't always translate well on social media. Sarcasm is often mistaken for earnest fecklessness. Legitimate earnestness is often mistaken for sarcasm. Cynicism is always seen for what it is, but your motives will always be misinterpreted, and though you were just reaching out to similarly minded cynics, you'll end up feeling more lonely and cynical. That being said, my status update was taken for exactly what it was: a public wound-licking. Within minutes of my message being posted, people started posting on my wall and sending me private messages, all offering heartfelt commiseration, understanding, and encouragement — some small poultice for the wound. But I was still hurt, and the injury was going to impede, at least temporarily, running's ability to fill the running-shaped hole. And that made it hurt even more.

I was winding down physio, and while my hips honestly did feel better, they were not up to 42.2K, or even 21.1K. I was running slowly and carefully, with a mind toward my new form — bum out (it feels like it's jutting out comically, like an old woman's bustle, but it's really not), leaning very slightly forward from the waist, chest out, multifidus muscles queued up by visualizing their elongation, treating the entire pelvic girdle as my suspension system (which it is) and keeping it loose and springy. Keeping that in the forefront of your mind on any run, let alone a full marathon, is taxing. It was going to be a long, slow rebuild. I considered myself lucky just to be able to get out there and run at all. Five or 6 kilometres at a time was a distance I could build on, but I wasn't about to push myself beyond that unnecessarily. I wasn't in training. I was learning how to run again, properly this time — and it was paying off. So, I was letting moderation be my byword. If I had really wanted to go limping through a full marathon, potentially injuring myself further, and maybe even anew in the process, I would have run Detroit.

But, there was more than injury and prudence stopping me.

Two weeks before the Detroit Half, I was out on a short, relaxed run with my friend Jane (an older sister of Elephant drummer, John). It was her first run of any kind in several weeks and one of my longer runs during the recovery process. On the run, we talked about how running Detroit was just completely out of the cards: irresponsible, dangerous, even. I was recovering from an injury; she was undertrained … it would be a disaster. Let's just run and be happy, we said. Good plan.

The very next day, Jane called. "I'm thinking about running Detroit," she said. "When we were running yesterday, it just felt so good. It motivated me to do it."

I listened and my chest tightened as Jane detailed how her sister Mary, who also had a running injury, had called from Port Perry and pleaded with Jane to run Detroit with her. Mary's husband, Dale, an experienced marathoner and ultra-runner, was in good race condition and would be way out in front. Mary didn't want to run alone and was looking for company along the race route. Both sisters were registered for the full marathon, but it was unlikely, they knew, that either of them would finish.

The moment I had foreseen with dread arrived, and my voice caught in my throat as she formally invited me to join them. "We'll just show up at the starting line on Fort Street in downtown Detroit and run whatever portion of the race our bodies allow us to run!" There would be periods of walking, she promised, lots of high-fiving with other runners and the people lining the streets, and ample time for no-pressure porta-john and water-station breaks.

Jane made a good case for just running the Detroit Free Press Marathon for fun: we'd get to run across the Ambassador Bridge at dawn, watching the sun rise over Windsor and Essex County; we'd, at least, get to experience the event and make use of the race packages we'd paid for with our registrations ... "Bobby," she said, "we can do this. *You* can do this!"

I realized the line had gone silent. Jane had stopped speaking, and I was just sitting there holding my breath, at a precarious loss for what to do, or say. Somehow, I hadn't prepared myself for this.

"You know there's that thing that if you don't run the race, you can't wear the shirt," Jane reminded me, softening her pitch, ever so slightly. "So, you might as well cross the border with us and get your shirt and your race kit. You paid for it ..."

She was right. There was definitely a part of me that wanted to pick up my race package, not only for the shirt, but to keep the option of running some portion of the marathon open. To collect your race package, which included your race bib, your official Detroit Free Press Marathon shirt, and any other swag that the event sponsors — shoe, apparel, and gear merchants — were pushing, you had to show up in person at the Fitness Expo at Cobo Center (now the TCF Center), a sprawling convention facility in downtown Detroit, on the Friday or Saturday prior to race day.

I would have to go to Detroit to collect my package. I would have to run around the city since the start and finish lines and the majority of the marathon course lies in Detroit ...

And therein lay my problem, because even if I was in prime condition; even if running the Detroit Free Press Marathon (or portions thereof) for fun had been something I really wanted to do, even if I just wanted to go pick up my fucking race package … all of this — ALL OF THIS — was precluded and made not only highly unadvisable but pretty much impossible by the fact that I might be going to jail. All my hips were stopping me from doing was running the marathon injury-free and optimally trained. No, as laid out in blunt detail by my lawyer, it was my current status as someone facing criminal charges that meant there was almost nothing so important that I should even consider crossing the border and risk being denied entry into the United States by U.S. Customs and Homeland Security. Not even my first full marathon.

Running had brought me to this.

CHAPTER TWELVE

SUPER-PATH SATURDAY

ON THE MORNING of May 31, 2014, Jennifer, the kids, and I went on a picnic in Willistead Park to celebrate the new asphalt paths that had been freshly poured there the previous day. By four o'clock that afternoon, I was sitting on a bench in City Hall Square, having just been released from jail.

With the exception of the two years I spent in Montreal, I have lived my entire life within a kilometre of Willistead Park. Aside from serving as a historical and cultural hub for the City of Windsor, the park — taking up an entire, oversized city block, and notable for its striking Tudor-Jacobean, Albert Kahn–designed manor house and gardens — also serves as the focal point for the Walkerville neighbourhood, with its rich whisky baron and rum-running lore, varying architectures, and stately, old trees.

I went there as a baby, pushed in my pram by my mother, my father snapping photos with his brand-new Canon 35 mm camera. I fell in love with books in the children's reading room during

Willistead Manor's tenure as a branch of the Windsor Public Library. Art in the Park weekends in early June through the '80s and '90s marked the unofficial start of summer. During my days at Walkerville Collegiate, the park became the lunchtime hangout in fair weather, the ideal place for smoking joints in all weather, an idyllic place to take your sketch board (and a joint) during senior art class … I grew up in Willistead Park. It was central to my neighbourhood. It was around the park's 1.2-kilometre wrought-iron and limestone pillar–fenced perimeter that I had walked, twice, instead of eating myself into a stupor following my cardiologist appointment, that sweaty and terrified day in late November 2012. The park, scene of so much "youthful" self-destruction, stuck around to play its role in saving my life.

Which is why, when the city announced plans for a new pathway system through the park, I was pleased. Where the city sidewalk around the park was in excellent condition, the interlocking brick path that bisected the park from north to south was in sorry disrepair. As a runner, as someone who believes in greater accessibility in public spaces, and as a lifelong Walkerville resident, I understood the need for the infrastructure upgrades and the accompanying drainage work that would protect Willistead Manor from flooding.

What I could not understand was why I came to feel so passionately about the paths and how I became embroiled in a situation that, prior to becoming a runner, I never would have been involved in. Clearly, the paths would be great for runners and the running community at large, but I wasn't about to start a Willistead Park running group, given my very conflicted relationship with group running. And running often took me far from Walkerville, so paved pathways in a neighbourhood park would have little overall impact on my running. I cared about my community but having spent fifteen years covering local news, I was loath to become one of those cranks who become overly and very vocally invested in local politics. Simply put, had you suggested to me at any time prior to the fall of 2013 that the new pathways in Willistead Park would become in any way significant in my life, become a symbol of my public persecution and of my very freedom, my response would have been dubious, at best. But that was before I'd heard of a group called Save Willistead Park!

Save Willistead Park! (exclamation point, theirs) was a rabid, near cult-like subsect of the entrenched Windsor history-buff scene, comprised of an awkward array of staunchly conservative, old-money Walkervillians, champagne socialists, radical environmentalists, and clueless reactionary glommers-on. The sole reason for the group's existence was to block any motion or work order that would make the park more widely accessible and user friendly. In the minds of the group's members, any such changes would threaten the sanctity of their off-leash dog-walking klatches and the group delusion that, because they lived nearby, the park belonged to them exclusively.

When the preliminary excavation and laying of the gravel bed for the pathways began, the Save Willistead Park! crowd lost their collective minds, called for an immediate halt to the work and the immediate undoing of the work that had been done. In press releases to traditional media outlets and online, they misrepresented the nature of the work, calling the pathways "industrial thoroughfares," "parking lots," and the "Willistead racetrack," all terms that were eventually supplanted by the stunningly drab coinage "super-paths."

A Save Willistead Park! Facebook group was created. The primary administrator of the group, and the strident spirit behind the whole Save Willistead Park! movement was none other than Sandra Voorhees, the very person who for two years had struggled to control my access to the lobby and front entrance to the *Windsor Star* building.

Since those days, we had been re-introduced to each other by mutual friends and acquaintances on a couple of occasions. At the time of one such encounter, I inscribed my second book of poetry to her. She was buying it at the urging of a former creative writing student of mine, who just happened to be her friend. She had a curious look on her face as I signed the book. I mentioned that we had worked together at the *Windsor Star* several years prior. Although she pretended not to know me, to have no recollection of our ever having worked together and been locked in a pitched battle of wills, unwritten corporate policy, and workplace culture, I always suspected she was demurring in her own strange-making way — like she was a bit blown away by the poetry, or something. What I'm trying to establish here is that Sandra Voorhees had occasion to know me well enough to know that I lived in Walkerville and would probably like to have some input on the plans for the new pathways. Indeed, she chose to invite both Jennifer and me to take part in the Save Willistead Park! Open Discussion Group on Facebook.

When Jennifer and I arrived at the group's page, we were both under the impression that anyone who was interested in "saving" Willistead Park would surely, like us, be in favour of the proposed pathways and drainage work, without which the park would fall into disrepair and become an inhospitable mire. What we found was a site that made clear that, in the eyes of the group, "saving" the park meant something else entirely. Also meaning something else entirely was the label, "Open Discussion Group," as the group's messaging was nothing but an open cesspool of anti-super-path rhetoric. Anyone in favour of the pathways was blocked, their comments deleted.

A public meeting with city councillors and planners, to be held in Willistead Manor, smack in the middle of the contested park, was scheduled for a blustery November night. Jennifer decided she was going to attend the meeting, to speak in favour of the pathways. I decided I was going for a run.

I arrived home first. I was stretched, showered, and changed, and pacing around the house, fighting the urge to walk down to the manor, when Jennifer returned, upset.

"It's a good thing you went for a run," she said, taking off her coat and tossing it over a chair. "You would have punched someone in the face." She went on to detail an evening of jeers and being shouted down by Save Willistead Park! demonstrators who were out in force for the public meeting. "You had to give your address at the microphone before speaking, and when I said Moy Avenue, a bunch of old men yelled that Moy Avenue isn't Walkerville, and whenever I tried to speak, they would interrupt me and make fun of me ..."

She was right. I definitely would have snapped one of these broken-down old Walkerville socialites over my knee like a mildewy log.

"I wish I was in good enough shape; I would have gone for a run with you," she said, exasperated.

And I felt doubly like shit: I hadn't been there to defend my wife against a bunch of drooling coots with their popped collars and gin-blossomed noses, the scions of the Save Willistead Park! scene and their over-powdered, gossip-mongering wives unsteady over their heels and under several drafts of gimlet; and I was the reason she wasn't able to enjoy the escapist benefits of running away from people like that. Though they were hard to get away from.

In my fifteen years in newspapers, I have never seen a local, grassroots group get as much ink as Save Willistead Park! There wasn't a print, broadcast, or web-based media outlet in the city that wasn't feasting on a steady diet of Sandra Voorhees's bizarre and emotionally overwrought opinions about the park's history and architecture and what she saw as the City of Windsor's failure to consult with her and her ilk. The war of words raged in letters to the editor and comment threads on social media through the winter and into the spring. In a story that appeared on a local online news site in May, more than two months after the city's decision to move ahead with the work in the park regardless of the protests, Sandra bemoaned the future of picnicking in the park, saying the very thought of picnicking within sight of an asphalt pathway being used by rollerbladers, cyclists, and people out for a walk ... It was simply too much for her to bear; and to make it known, she announced a "Walk for Willistead" slated for May 31.

○ ○ ○

The day before the anti-super-path protest walk, Jennifer arrived home in a state of excitement: "I just drove past Willistead," she said, wide-eyed. "They're done! The pathways are done!"

Jennifer was still detailing what she had observed on her thirty-second drive-by as I was hopping into a pair of running shorts and lacing up my New Balances. Arriving at the park's front gate on Niagara Street a few minutes later, I beheld the truth with my own eyes: it had all happened in a matter of hours over the course of that fine afternoon. There was no caution tape or signage; people were already strolling freely up and down the paths. I can't say for sure that I was the first runner to hit them, but I like to think so.

The pavement glittered like black, diamond-encrusted velvet. I ran with a joyful abandon — every step savoured, every squirrel and dog encountered treated with maximum *bonhomie*, every child and adult hailed from a distance and greeted with my standard "Hullo." I ran two clockwise laps around the park, exiting for a quick jaunt through the neighbourhood before re-entering the park for a turn along the freshly paved western arm of the pathways, and then heading home. A brisk thirty-minute 5K — about 2 kilometres of it happening on fresh Willistead Park asphalt.

Later that night, a friend messaged me to say there was much rending of virtual clothes and gnashing of digital teeth on the Ye Olde Save Willistead Park! Facebook group page, that I was missing out on a real chance to troll the crap out of the old guard while they were down and vulnerable. But I just wanted to maintain that good feeling of running on my neighbourhood's new paths through the night. And it was a good night. I slept the sleep of a sober runner: tired and peaceful. Their outrage, I told myself, was not as important as my serenity.

○ ○ ○

I woke up the next morning with the idea that we should go, as a family, to Willistead Park for a picnic. I was willing to push my long Saturday run back to later in the day in order to celebrate the successful installation of the asphalt pathways. It was important to show the Save Willistead Park! picnic authorities that it was, in fact, still possible to enjoy a picnic while an asphalt path meandered nearby through the grass.

"What if we run into that protest?" Jennifer said. "I don't want there to be a scene, especially with the kids there." She was also worried about the preparations for Jonah's birthday party (he had turned nine earlier in the week), which was happening later that afternoon. As well, Nathanael had a baseball practice and Thomasin was due to attend a birthday party for one of her friends — it was a Saturday with a lot of moving parts.

"We will be home in plenty of time, and I will help prep for the party. I can get Thomasin to her party and Nathanael to baseball," I reassured her while I raided the fridge and cupboards and poured what remained of that morning's coffee into a Thermos. I grabbed the novel I was reading, a book of poetry, my notebook, my fountain pen, put it all in a large picnic hamper, and with a collapsible camping chair slung over my shoulder, we set out for Willistead Park.

We found a nice plot of grass beneath a blossoming tree, near the freshly paved pathway, not far from the park's main gate on Niagara Street. We ate, the boys played catch, Jennifer and Thomasin alternated playing with a hula hoop and reading in the grass, and I read and enjoyed my coffee in my folding chair.

About a dozen protestors milled about on the driveway inside the park gate, about one hundred metres from our picnic spot. They carried placards that proclaimed such inanities as "Pave Roads Not Parks" and other inevitable and clumsily worded takes on Joni Mitchell's "pave paradise/parking lot" trope, and the idiotically confusing "We Love Grass."

To mark the occasion, I fired off a series of wry status updates and tweets, loosely livestreaming our picnic and mocking the insipid protest. A friend of ours, local lawyer of note and fellow poet Peter Horvat, happened on our picnic. Peter was enjoying the path as much as I was, and while the kids played, Jennifer, Peter, and I discussed the ridiculous impotence of the protest as it continued its stupefying clockwise vigil around the park. No attempt was made to engage them, as the whole point was to be as blithe, unencumbered, and serene as possible. It was a beautiful Saturday in May; we were having a family picnic, and the rest of day of birthdays and baseball still lay ahead of us.

With the picnic winding down, Jennifer decided she would take all three of the kids with her while she went shopping for supplies for Jonah's party. I opted to stay behind and enjoy the rest of the morning with my book and the still-well-topped Thermos of coffee. We agreed that I would be home in time to drop Nathanael off at his baseball practice.

At some point, the protest's numbers dwindled until just two remained — Sandra Voorhees and another woman — and I saw them entering the park through the main gates. They were too far away for me to hear what they were saying, but they carried in their arms all the placards that the Save Willistead Park! faithful had carried with them that day, standards to their obstinacy and pique. Mere feet from the intersection of the manor house's broad, curving driveway and the super-path trailhead, a newly installed garbage receptacle stood like a green sentinel droid. Sandra and her cohort stuffed one of their signs angrily into the receptacle's mouth and threw the other signs on the grass at the foot of the garbage bin. They then waved their arms dismissively, sick to death of the entire Willistead experience, and quit the park through the main gate.

I sat there in my chair, taking in what I had just witnessed. I finished my coffee and screwed the lid back on the Thermos. I folded up our picnic blanket and slipped it, along with my books and the leftover apples and cheese, into the picnic bag. I folded up my chair and slinging it over my shoulder in its sleeve, proceeded north down the fresh path toward the pile of discarded signs.

I knew that if I wasn't going to be part of the solution then I was part of the problem. I couldn't very well take offence to the littered protest signs and then walk away, leaving them there for somebody else to take care of. I gathered up the signs, wooden stakes and all — there were maybe five or six in total — and set out walking. I knew where Sandra lived because I ran by her house on a regular basis, and I often encountered her walking her two small dogs in and around Willistead Park. From the gates of the park, looking east down Niagara Street, I could see her house, no more than two hundred metres away. Her garbage was going home.

At my heaviest, I would have been paralyzed by fear at the thought of a possible confrontation. The very thought of walking 200 metres down the road to someone's house would have stopped me from going through the exertion of bending down to pick up the litter. But I was no longer an obese coward. This was the

225-pound Bob Stewart: a man emboldened by the confidence-boosting endorphins, potency, and litheness gained through running; a man who ran half-marathons; a man who could control his appetites. A man of solutions! A man of action! A man gently placing discarded protest placards on the porch of a woman's historic townhouse, arranging them in such a way that she couldn't fail to discover them the next time she stepped outside.

I was standing on the sidewalk in front of the Voorhees townhouse, snapping a few photos of my handiwork and posting them to Facebook and Twitter, being sure to tag our city councillor who had stooped to give Save Willistead Park! credence — to show him how they treated their beloved park once the battle was lost — when a voice called out to me:

"Hello? Excuse me? What are you doing? Do I know you?" It was Sandra Voorhees in her flower-print housedress, two small shih tzus on leashes nosing around her ankles.

"Hey, Sandra, it's Bob Stewart. We've met before. We used to work together at the *Windsor Star*. Anyway —"

"Excuse me — I don't know you! What are you doing? What is your business here? This is private property."

"Anyway, I was in the park having a picnic and I saw your impotent little protest and I also saw you littering, so I'm just bringing your garbage back to you so you can dispose of it properly. And, by the way, this isn't private property, this is a city sidewalk."

"Excuse me, sir, I have no idea who you are or why you are standing on my property, but you need to leave. You are frightening me."

I turned and started for home, crossing the street to give her and her dogs a wide berth. "Just don't litter in the park anymore, you fucking hypocrite," I said, fully planning to leave it at that.

But she started screaming. It was around lunchtime on a beautiful Saturday in late May. People were out tending to their lawns and gardens, reading, chatting on their porches … We immediately had a large audience.

"Help!" she shrieked. "This man is stalking me! I don't know this man! He followed me home from the park!"

"Sandra, we used to work together —"

"Help! This man is following me!"

I was laughing when I reached the other side of the street, where a man sat on the steps in front of his townhouse, smoking a cigarette.

Sandra saw him sitting there, too, and she called out to him: "Chad! Chad! This man is bothering me. He followed me home."

"Don't worry about it, Chad," I laughed. "I was just dropping off some garbage and now I'm on my way."

The man stood up from his stoop. He was wearing a dirty white T-shirt, jeans, work boots, and a ball cap. Everything was flecked with white paint and drywall spackle, including his hands. He flicked his cigarette in a wide arc across his lawn as he cut a direct path toward me. "What was that, fuckface?"

"This has nothing to do with you," I said. "I returned some litter to Sandra here, I'm on my way home and —"

"Where is it you fucking live? You're not from around here. What's your business in Walkerville?"

"Listen, I think you've got the wrong idea here. I just want Sandra to throw out her own garbage. It doesn't involve you."

By this time, Sandra was literally wringing her hands at Chad's elbow. Manic and breathless, she kept up a harridan's litany of complaints against me: how she didn't know me though I seemed to know her; how I had followed her home from the park; and, hilariously, how I had told her my name and it was "Robert Earl Jones" (I hadn't told her my name was Robert Earl *anything*. Although she messed up the last name, she knew me by both my given names).

I continued down Niagara, headed west for home, Sandra and Chad trailing a few feet behind me, Chad demanding to know where I lived and why I was in his neighbourhood.

"What is your business in Walkerville?" he kept demanding.

"I've lived here for forty years," I said. "Right here in this neighbourhood. That's my business here, *Chad*. It's not a private, gated community. Anyone can come and go as they please."

"I've never seen you before," he kept saying. "You're not from here."

By this time, Sandra and Chad had been joined by an older gentleman with a long white beard who was being pulled down the street by two hound dogs on chains. A posse.

"Find out where he lives, Chad," Sandra mewled at his elbow.

"Yeah, we'll find out where you live," Chad parroted. "We're going to follow you and find out where your shitbox house is, and when I do, you better hope you don't have kids or dogs around —"

I turned and put my finger in his face: "I gave you the opportunity to stay out of this back there, and now you're talking about following me home and making threats against my family and property? If I were you, *Chad*, I would get my ass back to that front porch and smoke some more cigarettes before you get yourself hurt. I'm not going to tell you again: you're not following me home."

While walking, I fired off another status update/tweet, stating I was now being followed home by the founder of Save Willistead Park! and some of her supporters, which included a pack of hounds. They were still on my tail half a block later when I stopped in front of the home of some of my oldest friends in the world: the Graysons. Sean, of course, had been the guitarist in Elephant. His father, Dr. George Grayson, still lived in the family home, a large Tudoresque manor in the heart of Olde Walkerville. My pursuers held back, forming a perimeter as if I was going to detonate the remains of my luncheon. *Should I just keep walking and hope my pursuers get bored? Do I break into a run, collapsible lawn chair, picnic hamper, and all, and do a Billy-from-Family-Circus-style tour of the neighbourhood, leaving the Save Willistead Park! posse winded and unable to follow my insipid parkour?*

From the street, I'd spotted a car on the parking pad at the rear of George's house. It appeared someone was home. Opting for safe harbour and a chance to let the situation subside, I walked up the flagstone path. I could hear Sandra Voorhees imploring someone to call the police as it was clear I was about to commit unlawful entry. "Why is he going to George Grayson's house?" she kept asking the two people with her, in turn. "He doesn't know George. We should call the police — look! He's knocking on the door. We can see you! What is your business in Walkerville?!"

It was going to be a wonderful moment when my knocks were heeded, and the door opened and I was welcomed into the home with open arms. But no one was coming to the door. I cupped my hands to the glass. All was still. I cut across the lawn and circled around to the back of the house. I could still hear them calling from the road, telling me there was nowhere to hide and that they were going to call the police and have me arrested for trespassing, as I rang the doorbell at the side door in vain. I moved around to the very back of the house and sat down at George's old picnic table. It was clear no one was home.

I could call Jennifer and tell her she needed to postpone the errand-running and drive down George's alley and pick me up behind his house. It was a good plan: easy, family-based, effective. But it also struck me as really emasculating — a grown man calling for his wife because some people were following him home. There was the WPD option. Sandra Voorhees, Chad, and the Hound Handler had even suggested it themselves. At the rate this was going, a visit from the police would be a welcome addition to this sad little tableau: a grown man sitting forlornly at a picnic table — alone, vexed, too proud to call for help. Surely the police had better things to do, actual criminals and miscreants to catch, women and children to protect …

I pulled my phone out of my pocket. A fresh reply to one of my posts popped up. It was from Matt McNeil, inquiring after my well-being: *I saw that last post. Are they still following you home? Do you need a hand?*

I'm good right now, I typed. *But if this guy named Chad gets too close, he's going to get a punch in the head.*

And that, really, in a nutshell, was it. I was a grown man; I was in the best shape of my life. What alcohol and overeating had slowly taken away, running had restored in a matter of months. Not just muscle tone, not just cardiovascular endurance. But balls. Why was I seeking refuge like a coward? I wasn't laying low so much as I was hiding from two senior citizens, a pair of shih tzus, two sway-backed beagles, and a feckless, spackle-flecked fellow named *Chad*. The police had better things to do than come escort me home; my wife and kids were better off not knowing that their husband and father, their protector and champion, was afraid to walk, as was his right, to his home because some people were being mean to him.

I stood up from George's picnic table, picking up the picnic hamper and lawn chair, and headed back out to the street. I had been doing my civic duty and was now being harassed. Cowering in obesity, I had for too many years been too afraid to defend myself and to speak out on behalf of others. Things were different now. I certainly wasn't going to lead them to our home, so the plan, if necessary, was to start my long Saturday run a bit early; invite my pursuers to keep up if they were able. Maybe these super-paths *would* lead to the formation of a running group?

Though the street was empty of angry mobs when I peered out from George's side lot, it wasn't long after I had crossed Niagara Street to the side with a city sidewalk that I realized the foreshortened wrought-iron bars of the Willistead Park fence had formed a black wall, preventing me from seeing Sandra, Chad, and a new person — the dark-haired woman who had littered on the park grounds with Sandra — standing in the mouth of the park's main gates. (No sign now of the Hound Handler.) Their smartphone cameras were out.

Chad came stomping across the street in his work boots, holding a smartphone in a hot pink case out in front of him. "The tables have turned!" he bellowed. "I am making a citizen's documentation video of your transgressions! Please state your name and address for the camera!" he commanded, exuding officious bluster. "State your name and address for the camera, sir!" he screamed, holding the camera so close to my face that any image would have been completely out of focus, blocking my vision in the process as I continued to walk backwards out into the intersection of Niagara and St. Mary's Gate.

I stopped there in the middle of the road. Chad, still shoving his smartphone in my face, Chad screaming at me for information, his cigarette breath and spittle hot against my cheeks. Sandra Voorhees and the other dark-haired woman (in her own floral housedress) began flanking me, moving beyond the limits of my poor peripheral vision, both of them shouting instructions at Chad, who I now stood face to face with in the intersection.

To be honest, it was the cigarette breath and the incoherent yelling that brought me to the tipping point, that was the catalyst for my effort to put an end to this ridiculous and rapidly escalating situation. I put my lung power to use, roaring some unrepeatable threat in Chad's face, startling him backwards and making him bring his hands up in front of his face in fright. Then I slapped the smartphone out of his hand, sending it sailing into the curb. And then I cocked my right hand and popped Chad in the mouth. His head snapped back, and he made an unintelligible sound. His legs went wobbly, and he stumbled around a bit, holding his hands down toward the ground as if to ward it off. And then, with a thin line of blood running down his chin, he started to cry.

"I warned you," I said. "Several times. I told you to back off."

Of course, he couldn't hear me because Sandra Voorhees was clutching her head and shrieking as if I had just cut Chad in half, from stem to stern, with a sword. I adjusted my baggage and turned to walk the rest of the way home in relative peace, as Chad began digging frantically in his pocket, producing a second phone. He held it up like a talisman. "Now you've done it," he said. "That's assault! That is assault! I'm phoning the police. You're going to jail!" He dialed the three digits on his phone with great purpose.

Run, I told myself. *This is why you train. This is why you walked twice around the park. This is why this is happening right here, right now.* But where weight and immobility would have prevented me from making my escape in the past, now it was pride and — as I laughed in Chad's face, calling him a sissy and mocking his crushed bravado — I realized, even cruelty. I wasn't about to run like a coward. I had confronted adversity head on, and now I was going to be on my leisurely way. As I continued in the general direction of home, Chad hustled along behind me, stanching his mouth with his shirt, giving a description to dispatch. Sandra and the dark-haired woman barked out directions as I turned north on Chilver Road, as if I was speeding away in a roadster and not strolling blithely down the street.

When I heard Chad sign off, I was walking in front of King Edward Public School, the school I had graduated from some twenty-six years previous, the school all three of my children attended, the school I had for years been afraid to accompany them to because I didn't want to embarrass them with my weight. But now that I knew the police were on their way, I wanted to stick around and get this straightened out. So, I stopped, which froze

Chad in his tracks, and slid my collapsible lawn chair out of its nylon sheath, opened it up, and parked myself under one of the trees lining the school property. Chad kept his distance, pacing like an angry old man in a comedy, while Sandra and the other woman circled around to the far end of the block to hem me in. In a matter of minutes, a police cruiser turned up the street and made a slow approach. I stood up from my chair, smiled at Chad, who skittered off to join the women, and raised my hand to hail the cruiser.

The police cruiser slowed to a stop at the curb and two young officers got out, adjusting their belts and surveying the various parties. A few people had gathered on the sidewalk and porches across the street. One of the officers asked me what the problem was.

I pointed down the street to where Chad stood. "Thanks for responding so quickly, officer," I said. "That man there has been following me for several blocks, making threats against my family and property. I asked him repeatedly to stop following —"

"Why is he bleeding?"

"Well, he got too close, and I punched him in the face."

The words were hardly out of my mouth when I was grabbed on both sides and thrown heavily against the back of the cruiser. My hands were twisted behind me, and I felt the cuffs going on as one of the officers told me I was being placed under arrest for assault.

Our picnic hamper was dumped out on the cruiser's trunk deck, the police officers seizing on my black fountain pen as an article of drug paraphernalia. I told them it was an expensive pen as one of them unscrewed the cap, sniffed it, unscrewed the barrel from the section, looking for the chamber that contained the weed or rocks they fully expected to find. When they didn't find what they wanted, they asked how I happened to be in the possession of such a fine writing instrument. I told them I bought it at a pen store in Toronto, which opened up a whole other thread of questioning about my travels and whereabouts in recent days, which eventually led to them asking for my ID and checking my address as given on my driver's licence with dispatch. They also sniffed suspiciously at the coffee in my Thermos and dumped it, callously, into the gutter. The two constables began interviewing Chad, Sandra, and the woman who was wearing a house dress. A crowd was forming on the street.

One of the young constables asked if there was anyone I wanted to call. He fished my phone out of my pocket and dialed Jennifer's cell number for me, and for the second time that hour, someone was holding a phone up to my face. He dutifully held the phone to my ear while I talked to my wife.

In the way of husbands and wives the world over, she could tell something was wrong as soon as she answered the phone. "There's been an incident," I said. I told her that I wasn't hurt, but that I had been arrested and was being taken downtown.

"Why did you want to go on that picnic at all?" she said through clenched teeth. "I told you there would be trouble. You *knew* there would be trouble."

"No. I didn't want this," I said, leaning slightly into the phone as the constable who was holding it to my ear lost focus. "I don't have much time here."

"Okay, what should I do?" she said through her tears.

"Call a lawyer," I said. "And don't tell the kids."

In my years in newspapers, I've seen actual suspected murderers, surrendering to cops in a dive bar, be gently placed in the back of a cruiser for the ride downtown. But I was deemed far too dangerous to be placed in the back of a cruiser with the only thing separating me from the two downy-cheeked rookies in the front seat being an inch of bullet-proof Plexiglas. The paddy wagon had been summoned to the scene, and soon enough, it came trundling down Cataraqui Street, coming to an angled stop in the intersection with Chilver as if it were pulling up on an intense siege situation.

Chad stuck around for a front-row seat to my being hauled away. He was the cock of the walk now that I was in handcuffs. I was surprised at how close he was allowed to get to me as I was marched down to the paddy wagon. He stood there, chirping told-you-sos and promises of seeing me in court from his swollen, bloody lips.

I mouthed one final, tender kiss in his direction as I was taken around the back of the vehicle.

Paddy wagons have come a long way from the bleak, dented, piss-, vomit-, and shit-reeking cubicles film, television, and noir fictions had conditioned me to expect. Looking into the rear-entry maw of the "prisoner transport" section of the vehicle, I was struck by the fact that the stainless steel-clad interior was spotlessly clean, gleaming even; perhaps some poor civilian lackey who toiled in the bowels of the WPD HQ was made to polish it at gunpoint every night. I was also struck by all the things I was likely to be struck by or be struck against once we were in motion: a seemingly capricious number of angled steel bulkheads on the walls and ceiling of the vault-like cell. The ceiling was too low to stand up under, so it was necessary to sit on one of the stainless steel clad benches that lined each side.

I was helped up the stairs and sat down on the bench and turned to my captors. "Can't help but notice there're no seat belts back here," I said, as the doors were closed in my face.

I tell you, you've never seen your city, town, or corner of our great dominion until you've seen it through the grate-covered window in the back of a prisoner-transport vehicle. You can try to brace yourself by pressing your shoulders into the wall behind you and planting your feet wide against the floor and bench opposite. But without restraints, aside from the ones holding your hands behind your back, and without any friction between your clothing and the polished steel cladding, and with a driver determined to see how many times he can throw you into the angled steel bulkheads in the small chamber — stomping on the brakes at stop signs, then gunning it from dead stops, taking turns with vicious abandon … It was a bruising trip downtown.

The truck went down several ramps into the bowels of Windsor's police headquarters and came to a stop on a large, well-lit, underground parking pad. Armed police officers appeared through a large steel door and stood, ready for action, a few defensive paces from the back of the vehicle.

I did my best to look blasé and nonchalant when the driver came around and opened the doors, as if I'd been enjoying the relaxing ride and the bucolic vistas of the downtown core. I was led through the steel door and onto a service elevator, which rose through the building. When the doors opened I was standing before a large, curved desk in what was clearly the prisoner-processing area. A tired-looking senior constable–type looked over some paperwork and logged all the possessions I came in with — my wallet, keys, and phone, and your typical bandit's tool kit of collapsible lawn chair, empty Thermos, crumpled cheddar cheese packaging, apple, notebook, fountain pen, works of contemporary fiction and poetry. Then they took my belt and my running shoes.

There are over two hundred thousand people in Windsor, but all the City of Roses had to offer that day was a drunk moaning through a hangover and a poet who punched a guy in the face. I sat on the cement bench and looked around my cell: aside from the bench, there was a stainless-steel commode unit, and graffiti — detailing who was innocent, who was guilty, who sucked whose dick, and who was a whore — etched into the Plexiglas rivetted as a barrier over the bars.

I pulled my stockinged feet up off the slip-resistant concrete floor, closed my eyes, and did some square breathing. There was no use panicking. There was no use weeping. Everything that happened, I knew, had happened for a reason. And as I sat there, cross-legged on the concrete bench in the holding cells of the Windsor Police Department jail, I was not scared; I was not worried; I was not under duress. Rather, I was filled with a feeling of being greatly and inordinately blessed. I was filled with a peace and serenity: I knew why I had struck another man, knew that I was in the wrong, and though I did not know what was going to happen to me next, knew that I was going to be taken care of, that I was supported and loved, and that I was sober and was further removed from a drink than I had been when I woke up that morning.

That this was my first time in a jail cell was, alone, testament to just how blessed I was. With the exception of the days following my mother's death and funeral services in 2006, I can think of few times when I felt closer to the God of my understanding than I did sitting there in jail. It looked like I was going to miss my long run, so I was going to have to get my meditation in somewhere. This was quiet and afforded me as much privacy, outside of the drunk sleeping it off in a cell across the way, as a man with three kids is likely to get on a weekend.

At some point during my stay, the kindly, older cop who I first encountered at the processing desk came and passed two cheeseburgers and two juice boxes through the meal slot. A word about these cheeseburgers: clouds of cheeseburger-scented steam escaped as the cellophane was ripped open. What lay inside was something to behold: smashed flat, as if prepared with blunt instruments, they were condiment free (possibly even foodstuff free), but, in saying that, I have eaten worse.

The kindly old cop returned later and took me for fingerprinting and documentation in a glassed-in identification laboratory. My inked fingers were rolled on a digital pad; my retinas were scanned; I was made to swab the inside of my cheeks for DNA (just in case I turned up in Interpol as one of the world's foremost neighbourhood miscreants); I sat before the camera and had my mugshot taken. It was all very cordial and lasted maybe ten minutes before I was returned to my cell.

I urinated with great caution, taking care where I placed my stockinged feet around the base of the commode. It occurred to me I had no idea how this worked. I had no idea whether I was going to be home for supper or asking for a blanket at 3:00 a.m. I had no way of telling the time and was trying to keep a mental concept of how many minutes had passed since I last had a definite sense of the hour. I kept expecting the door to the cell block to open and see someone coming to bail me out. Who would it be: my wife, pallid with worry, her father standing with her, bankrolling my freedom; or, God forbid, my father, bewildered and disappointed, expecting to be presented with a soiled, booze-reeking disgrace of a son, and glad, for once, that my mother — who once warned me that if I ever ended up in jail, to not bother calling because they would not come to get me — was not there to see this. But whenever I heard voices in the corridor beyond the steel-and-reinforced-glass door of the holding cells, it was just police and staff, chatting, laughing, going about their business. The man in the cell across from me moaned and fussed in his inebriation. And no one came for me.

Loneliness will, eventually, erode some of your spiritual resolve. Running has taught me this.

The Promise to Appear I signed when they eventually came to get me from my cell had me agreeing to show up in court on the morning of July 3, 2014, to face the charges of one count of mischief and one count of assault, both deeds contrary to the Criminal Code of Canada.

I was given a clear plastic bag that contained my personal effects. I slipped on my shoes and didn't bother with my belt. I slung the collapsible lawn chair and vinyl picnic bag over my shoulder and followed the kindly, older cop down a few flights of concrete stairs before coming to a plain, steel door. Before he pressed down on the bar to open it, the old cop asked what the rest of my day was going to be like. I honestly didn't know. I don't remember what I told him. When the door swung open, it was not into the darkness of night, nor into a dingy alley that I stepped, but rather into the sunlight of midafternoon, onto the sidewalk on Goyeau Street.

I turned to the cop and asked him the time. He glanced at his watch: "Quarter after four," he said, before bidding me adieu and closing the door softly.

I walked around the corner to the cenotaph at City Hall Square. I took a seat on a bench. The 225-pound version of me could walk the 2.5 kilometres home. Hell, the 225-pound version of me was more than capable of running that distance in twelve minutes. But those were fleeting thoughts. I had nothing in the tank. I was at a physical and spiritual low tide. I pulled my phone out of my pocket and called Jennifer.

I was still sitting on the bench by the cenotaph when she pulled up at the curb. Her cheeks were hot with tears.

CHAPTER THIRTEEN

IMMANENT JUSTICE

"WHY COULDN'T YOU just let it go?" she cried.

"I didn't want them to win," I said.

"The pathways are in!" she said. "They'd already lost!"

I had no defence against this. There was nothing I could say.

The night of Super-Path Saturday, upon arriving home — Jonah's birthday having gone off without a hitch without my help, the kids having been informed that I had gone off to run some errands and told some other plausible lies that covered for my daylong absence — Jennifer and I sat on the porch. We spoke in hushed tones. She cried a bit — partly out of anger at my recklessness, out of anger at herself for not being there to hold me back, to calm that savage side of me that I didn't like her to see, but largely out of anger at what I had gone through to end up in jail with charges hung around my neck. There was also the fear of how those charges and a criminal defence were going to affect our family budget. This all happened just days after Jennifer convinced me to resign from the newspaper. Just when it had seemed my journalism career was wrapping up as neat as a bow, I had to go and punch a guy in the face.

"I don't know how we're going to do this," she said, staring off across the street, unable to look at me. "How much does a lawyer even cost? I'm afraid to even tell me parents. They could maybe help, but what am I going to say, 'We need thousands of dollars to keep Bob out of jail for beating a man up in the street'?"

"I didn't beat him up," I said, quietly. "It punched him, once. In self-defence. There's a big difference."

She didn't want to hear it. "Can you call the newspaper and see if you can have your old job back? What if you end up in jail? What if we lose the house? What if you can never work again? What will I tell the kids? What will they tell their friends — 'My dad's in prison. He beat a guy up in the street because he really hates litterbugs'?"

She wasn't wrong. And I was totally at a loss to provide any answers or insight into why any of this was happening.

The lawyer Jennifer called that Saturday after receiving my phone call was Peter Horvat. We'd been talking to him in the park just minutes prior to things getting out of hand. The criminal defence lawyer Peter recommended was named Johnny Rydel. "He's an old English major — just like us!" said Peter. "He understands guys like you and me!" Peter clearly wasn't referring to us jointly as well-to-do lawyers, or criminals, so I could only assume he meant as poets.

I'd never met anyone who understood poets, including and especially other poets, but call Johnny Rydel I did, leaving what was probably a frantic and incoherent voicemail message in the hours following my release from the holding cells. Johnny called me back on the Monday, two days after the conflagration. His tone was avuncular, and his voice lacked urgency, which was reassuring. He asked me a bit about what had happened, a bit about my background, whether I was married, had a job, kids — whether I had a criminal past.

"No criminal past at all?" His laugh was tinged with disbelief.

"No, nothing," I said. "Parking tickets, a couple of speeding tickets. A police officer made us dump out a half-case of beer in the park in high school ..."

He seemed satisfied with this and invited me to come down to his office for a little chat. Like this phone call, he said, there would be no charge for our meeting. He said that if after our meeting I was interested in having him represent me in court — and there was certainly no pressure to do so — I would simply have to pay his retainer. He would then be my official representative in this matter. I didn't see any point in prolonging the search for legal representation. Here was a criminal defence attorney, recommended to me by a friend in the legal profession, calling me at home, and inviting me down for a chat in his office, gratis. On top of all that, he was a known fan of poetry. I told Johnny I would very much like to come down to his office for that chat. We arranged to do that the next day. Before we terminated the call, I needed to clarify something:

"Do I need to wear anything special tomorrow?" I asked. "Like a jacket or a tie?"

Dead silence from the other end of the line before a wry chuckle. "Wow, you really *haven't* done this before, have you?" His voice led me to believe he was impressed with my naïveté. "Let me tell you something, Robert," he said. "I have some of the lowest criminal types you can imagine in and out of my office on a day-to-day basis. You can wear whatever you want."

○ ○ ○

I met with Johnny in his office in a rambling Ouellette Avenue manor house a few days later. We talked about the particulars of the case. Based on my total lack of criminal record, Johnny seemed fairly certain that this was going to work out in my favour. "As far as I can see, it's a neighbourhood dispute that escalated, no one has been seriously injured, and there was no premeditation," he explained. I had done wrong, but I was lucky. The court, he said, was not going to spend too much time on this one.

The next day, I was back in Johnny's office with an envelope fat with $1,130 cash (all twenty-dollar bills, like a hardened criminal) drained from our family bank account and tucked into a bank deposit envelope. Our account was well into overdraft, but I'd retained my criminal defence.

Jennifer, through all of this, was maybe not as furious as most wives would be after picking their husbands up from jail downtown after the family picnic descends into fisticuffs and neighbourhood unrest. The drinking years had prepared her for this potentiality. Where running had quelled a lot of that latent rage, it had clearly given me greater confidence in my ability to protect myself.

As the summer wore on toward late July, I figured no major news was good news. Johnny would occasionally call to let me know that my matter before the courts had been once again put over by a judge. Johnny insisted this was a good thing: whenever you could buy time in an assault case, it worked in the defendant's favour, he said. It gave everyone a chance to cool down and move on. Although it tried my patience, I had to put my faith in Johnny's word.

I continued to run and train in preparation for the Detroit Full with reckless abandon. Not surprisingly, the running-shaped hole was difficult to reach, the path being cluttered with snippets of footage from what came to be known at Super-Path Saturday.

In August, the Crown Attorney's office said they were amenable to talking about a peace bond. Johnny gave me some homework: I was to gather up some character reference letters — written testimonials from friends and family attesting to my gentle nature and generous character, and my status as a community-minded family man, prominent local journalist, and writer of some regard. The Crown would take these letters into consideration when approaching the complainants about a peace bond. The catch in peace bond situations, though, is this: the complainants have to agree to the peace bond. The Crown can suggest it, but all the power in a peace bond solution lies with the complainant. "So, the better your letters," Johnny said, "the better your chances."

When I presented Johnny with my stack of letters two weeks later, he was pleased. It was an impressive docket of Windsorites, including doctors, lawyers, publishers, municipal politicians, well-known social activists, and sitting members of Parliament, all of whom saw me as something other than Walkerville's preeminent miscreant and degenerate alcoholic, which was the image the Save Willistead Park! crowd was pitching to the Crown. There wasn't a barrister in the Crown's office that could fail to at least acknowledge that there were some serious, socially aware heavy hitters represented in the correspondence. And if Johnny was buoyed by the letters, then I would try and be buoyed, too. There was light — and a light wrist slap — at the end of this dark stretch of bad road.

The reprieve was short-lived.

I ran as many kilometres as I could, keeping track of kilometres missed due to thunderstorm and tornado, until my body stopped me cold, and my physiotherapist said I was going to need a lot more than bad weather to fix my messed-up hip and get me to the start line in downtown Detroit.

It was a bad time to find myself shelved. Running hadn't exactly been the meditative release I counted on following the contretemps at the park gates, but at least it had been something — a salve for my fears and wounded pride. Because even though Johnny didn't seem worried, without the therapeutic outlet of running, I vacillated between cautious optimism and dread.

It was only once any hope of running the Detroit Full had been dashed that it occurred to me that training myself into disrepair in an attempt to run a marathon had provided a convenient excuse for the real reason I wasn't going to be running. Somehow, I had lost sight of the fact that crossing the border into the United States with a matter before the courts in the age of Homeland Security was not advisable. Johnny had counselled me against this at our first meeting.

Quite truthfully, I had fully expected the wheels of justice to have made their full and, for me, exonerating revolutions and to have had everything all wrapped up, charges dismissed, complainants and Crown attorneys alike reprimanded by a judge, well in advance of October 19, the day of the marathon. But as summer wore on and it hadn't come to pass, it became less and less likely that I was going to be able to cross the border to get to the starting line. Against both the Crown and my nagging injuries, it was an uphill battle. What it all came down to was this: healthy or hurt, confident in my training or terrified, it had pretty much been guaranteed from the moment I decided to punch a guy in the face (or was it when I decided to pick up someone else's garbage and make them responsible for it; or was it when I decided to go for a picnic in the park?) that I was not going to be running that race.

"That race has morphed into a white whale for you, my friend," said my running friend Anastasia. "I'm going to start calling you Ahab."

"Call me Ishmael," was my witty rejoinder, though the truly funny thing was that Anastasia had really hit at the heart of the matter with the harpoon of truth she fired into my ruddy-white flank.

The Detroit Free Press Marathon didn't represent a performance-based white whale. It wasn't an obstacle on the road to weight loss and increased health and fitness. You don't need to register for a race to go run your fool ass off. I'd proven that the previous October with the Me Press Half. In fact, lots of people lose weight running and never run or register for a single race of any kind. And it's not like I had delusions of what would happen in Detroit: I would run and struggle and complete the race in my own five-plus-hour way. No, the Detroit Free Press Marathon had become some kind of spiritual bugaboo, a chimera I could not run down, a quest that I could not finish. In fact, I could not ever make it to the starting line.

Two years of training for and failing to run Detroit can hardly be described as forming a pattern, but there was definitely something about me and this race, like it was not meant to be. Accepting that, accepting that this was not coincidence, that it was all happening the way my Higher Power wanted it to happen was humbling in a way I had not yet experienced. I could do battle with land-based leviathan for days, struggling against it, but my real adversary was, again, as always, me. It didn't matter how much I ran, nor how much time I spent in the meditative space of the running-shaped hole: I was still susceptible to self-sabotage at the hands of the worst parts of my character. The really maddening thing: it's the people who are always getting in their own way — people like me, going for picnics and winding up in jail — who would benefit from the spiritual experience of confronting the nemesis of a big run.

Looking back on that Sunday morning, when I lay in bed, avoiding any news of the marathon and hiding from the world at large while people bled from their nipples and ran their heart and lungs out on the streets of Detroit, was I hiding from the knowledge of the race, or was I hiding from knowledge of myself? Hiding from the knowledge that, despite eleven years of sobriety, a patient and loving wife and three beautiful children, a home, jobs, publishing contracts, my newly regained health, the ability to not only run but to train for a marathon, I still needed to punch a smaller, weaker man in the face to make sure he took me seriously; to make sure my ego was acknowledged and satisfied? For the record, I'm going to say both. Of course, if I was willing to lie at the border and risk deportation and the dreaded red brand of "Denied Entry" status, as well as possibly getting tossed into an American prison, it was all so tantalizingly close … On days like that Sunday, a day when it kind of feels like you've taken a shit in the running-shaped hole, I think it's perfectly okay, and even normal and rational, to hate yourself a little bit.

One of the things that had been affecting me so deeply was the tension I had unwittingly created between the close friends and confidants who knew the full story, and other close friends and confidants, including my own father and sister, who did not. My efforts to protect the people who stood to be hurt the most from the knowledge of what I had done had resulted in a two-tiered economy of truth based solely on my shame.

This was the real lesson to be learned from all of this: dealing with Sandra Voorhees and punching Chad (whose last name turned out to be Poupard) in the face had served a higher purpose. These events were showing me where I was at. Although there were a lot of things that were an improvement over not only the past eighteen months but the last decade, some four thousand days of sobriety as of that late-May morning, there was also definitely something amiss. Somewhere within the heterotopic space of running, there was something rotten. That interior place had found a locus in the real world: Willistead Park. Had running, maybe, led me astray, further inflated my sense of self, given me a dangerous confidence that brought with it a renewed willingness to engage people physically because I was no longer afraid of being unable to defend myself? Was I making up for all the lost opportunity to pound people who had poked fun at my weight when I was nearly four hundred pounds by coldcocking the first guy to not take the 225-pound version of me seriously? Doubtless, there were many who deserved it, but if I was supposed to be living a different life, one where I have a daily solution to the catastrophe of the self, a sober life that I committed myself to, and did my best to practise in all of my affairs ... What was I thinking? More importantly, what was I doing, or not doing?

As easy as it was to see the whole situation as overwhelmingly negative; to start wallowing in my own self-pity (beyond the one- or two-day wallow that I virtually insist upon when I am feeling particularly wounded or depressed); to start seeking comfort in stuffing my face; to stop running; to grab hold of the reins and start guiding the ship by willpower and wrong-thinking, I just kept running. I ran through Willistead Park the day after I was released from the holding cell. I started training for Detroit, a race I must have known, on some level, that I might not even get the chance to run. And I did this because I knew, thank God, that the problem was *not* other people, as much as I disliked them. The problem was, and always had been, *me*. And the solution for me is action — not in the form of confrontation and intellectual debate and social posturing and municipal politics ... but in running: running away from turmoil and self-will-run-riot; running toward the sober solution that saved my life, and on into the running-shaped hole. Because running had not led me astray; my will and my ego had.

○ ○ ○

In late October, Johnny called with some bad news. The Crown attorney had adamantly rejected even the suggestion of a peace bond as a way to settle the matter, refusing to even approach the complainants with the suggestion for their consideration and approval. Johnny was disappointed and apologetic; he even sounded a bit flustered and confused, unable to figure out why the Crown was so determined to get a conviction against someone with a clean record — a first-time offender — on such a minor assault and mischief charge. I agreed to meet with Johnny in his office the next day to discuss out next move.

"I think I figured out why they wouldn't do the peace bond," Johnny said, as I was ushered into his office. He tossed a sheaf of papers onto the desk in front of me, the file folder that had once held them splayed awkwardly beneath.

On top of the sheaf of papers was a printout of a screen capture of my social media post detailing being followed home by Sandra, Chad, et al., Matt McNeil's offer of assistance, and my promise to punch Chad Poupard in the head if he got too close to me.

"Did you write these things?" Johnny asked, chipper, genuinely interested.

"Why, does it hurt my case?"

"It certainly doesn't help!" he yelled, flipping through page after page of my scathing commentaries — most of which I thought had been deleted along with my generic support for the pathways — from the Save Willistead Park! social media feeds. All of it had been sent in duplicate to the Windsor Police by the Crown Attorney's office. I looked up at Johnny, who sat across from me, leaning back in his chair, staring me down, a mane of deep red curls and a bolo tie.

"I needed to know these things," he said, bemused. "I can't walk into court on your behalf and ask a judge to throw this matter out when there's a whole stack of paper floating around that shows, at the very least, a history of online harassment and a premeditated intent to assault someone."

I was stunned at the floating of the term *online harassment*. I launched into a vociferous defence of my tweets and postings as just me doing my job as a journalist; that one of my jobs as a newspaper editor was to satirize the local goings-on; that my reply to McNeil's query after my safety and well-being was nothing more than a statement of my intent to defend myself if certain parties did not back the fuck off.

"Judges tend *not* to buy the 'pre-emptive strike' defence," Johnny said.

What he had originally characterized as a worst-case-scenario peace bond situation, where I would never see the inside of a court-room and certainly not the inside of a prison cell, had taken an unexpected turn.

My legal defence had just become much more difficult. My initial retainer of $1,130 was no longer going to cut it. Johnny wasn't going to be able to breeze in and out of court on my behalf. Some more serious legal wrangling was going to be required. As well as an additional $2,500. We'd gone from a situation where Johnny was sure he could get the charges thrown out, to hoping for a peace bond, to looking at a mid-December court date and whether I was going to plead guilty or not guilty to the charges, thanks almost entirely to my not-helpful tweets and social media ramblings, obviously collected over a period of time and curated into a neat little document by Save Willistead Park! social media admins for just such an occasion.

I'd made my lawyer look like a fool, and he wasn't afraid to take it out on me. Which made me feel, rightly, like a total fucking idiot. One of the big takeaways from this whole ordeal: never forecast punching someone in the face on social media.

"We're going to have to get out ahead of this whole anger management issue you've got going on," Johnny said, returning to his more avuncular self. "Judges look very favourably on defendants who appear before them and are taking their charges seriously, taking steps to make sure it never happens again. I don't see you going to jail, but we have to be realistic here …"

I felt the onset of a panic attack at the edges of my vision.

"I think the best we can hope for now is a conditional discharge. You won't be convicted of a crime, but you will be given a period of probation during which you would be prohibited from leaving the country for some time, and you would be hit with weapons restrictions, which is neither here nor there, and you would be forced to enter a period of anger management. So, if we can show that you are doing this on your own volition ..."

Indeed, getting out in front of the whole "anger management" thing seemed like the kind of prudent, self-improving decision that a man — a poet — who deeply regretted punching a piece of shit in the face would make. And of course, Johnny knew a guy.

○ ○ ○

The guy I went to see was a social worker named Stephen J. Bruce.

Stephen was a large cask of a man, salt-and-pepper coiffed, with a walrus-style moustache, kind eyes, and a deep voice full of understanding. Johnny had updated him on my case, and he was familiar with the broad strokes of Super-Path Saturday. He said he would write a letter for the judge when we were done with our sessions, saying that I had "worked out my 'anger issues'" (he put big, sarcastic air quotes around the term).

"But that's really a secondary outcome of this process," Stephen said. "What the judge decides is beyond our control. What we can control, and what I'm here to do is help you find a way to avoid these situations in the future because, as I'm sure you are well aware, the world is full of people like Mrs. Voorhees and Mr. Poupard. More importantly, you need to come to terms with a situation that has really shaken you and, from what John tells me, made you lash out in a way that is very out of character."

Talking openly about personal struggles is not something that comes naturally. Not for me; not for most people. But ever since I figured out it was *good for me* — right around the time I stopped drinking and sought help for my alcoholism in my late twenties — I've benefitted greatly from sharing openly and honestly with others. It has become a crucial part of my sobriety, a crucial part of my life. The most important thing I've learned in sharing my troubles with others is that the better part of talking about your troubles is listening. So, when Johnny suggested I see Stephen as a way to show the Ontario Superior Court judge that I was taking proactive steps to prevent anything like a repeat offence from ever happening again, I was not only willing to do it, I looked forward to it.

We settled into our respective chairs, separated by a low table with our mugs of coffee and the obligatory box of tissues. Stephen asked me about my family background, upbringing, education, career, interests. I spoke about growing up in Walkerville, Jen and the kids, how I had left the *LaSalle Post* that summer. I told him about my running, and how I had once weighed nearly four hundred pounds; about my recovery from alcoholism and my continued commitment to a way of life that allowed me to be sober on a daily basis.

We talked about past instances of violence — everything from the schoolyard to the barroom. Stephen pointed out that just because it is not *totally* out of character to lose your temper and lash out in anger — and even though it can feel powerful and intoxicating to do so — doesn't mean we don't pay a heavy emotional and spiritual price when we do.

"Why don't you tell me what happened that day," he said, all calm and openness.

I told him the story: the day-long narrative that despite repeated retellings and near constant replay in my head for the past five months had not diminished one iota in its ability to get my blood up. I brought him right through to sitting on the porch following my release from jail, Jen's tears of anger, fear, and disappointment making tracks in the gloaming.

We sat in the silence for a few moments, before Stephen said, softly, "Sounds like a pretty terrible day."

I agreed that it had been. "Jen and the kids must've been worried," he said. I reached for a tissue.

"The kids still don't know," I said.

"No? Why is that?"

"Because we don't want them to know what I did; that I was arrested and spent the day in jail."

"Not very good behaviour, is it," he said.

That was the end of our first meeting.

○　○　○

In subsequent meetings, Stephen and I focused on my behaviour — how it affects my family, how it affects the standards I have for myself, particularly as someone with so much invested in living differently in sobriety. When Stephen asked what made me snap that day, what made me cause so much pain, I said I feared for my safety.

"Bullshit," Stephen said. "I'm not a cop, Robert. You don't have to tell me what you told *them*. You weren't scared for your safety. Why did you hit him?"

"He wasn't listening to me. He wasn't taking me seriously."

"He was disobeying you."

"Yes. I couldn't understand why he wanted to provoke me when it was pretty obvious that I could hurt him."

"But rather than feel sorry for him — maybe he's a sick person? — you punched him in the face."

"Yes. I felt, at the time, that he deserved it."

"You still feel he deserved it, no?"

"Yes."

"There's a big gap between feeling that someone deserves to be punished and being the person who believes himself responsible for punishing that person, isn't there?" He let that sink in. "Who made you responsible for punishment? Who made it okay for you to physically assault someone in the streets?"

I had no answers. Stephen asked me if I was familiar with the Swiss clinical psychologist Jean Piaget and his concept of *immanent justice*. I knew the name, but that's it. "Your sense of justice, Robert, is immature. It is tied to what are called 'just-world beliefs,' a child-like belief in a manageable and predictable world where every wrongdoing and every bad deed is met with an immediate punishment. You see the world in these black-and-white conditions. And when you see someone getting away with something that you, in your immature black-and-white way, see as unjust, you decide that you have to be the agent of that justice. That you are going to be the person who metes out the punishment that restores balance and harmony. Do you think you achieved that that day at the park?"

It wasn't difficult for me to jump to the conclusion that everything that was happening to me was punishment for the cumulative past deeds of my teens and twenties: my alcoholism, my drug use, my gluttony, my pride. I had not outrun these things. They had not disappeared from my system with sloughed off fat cells. No amount of 5K and 10K medals, race bibs, and commemorative running shirts and hats could absolve me of these things. They were alive and waiting for me to fail, so they could take me into the back alley of my psyche and finish the job. Whether I understood the concept of immanent justice or not made little difference to the fact that immanent justice was precisely the kind of justice I, at forty years old, still believed in.

I was not looking for a way out of it. I was looking for a way beyond it, to span that gap between maturity and immaturity, to know that justice had much broader, much more complex cause and effect connections than those understood inherently by children, to understand that I was not the agent of reward, or punishment, or even mercy. I just wanted to be a better man.

Sure, you can sober up, you can run off the weight, but if you pray for humility and the ability to accept life on life's terms, you had better buckle up. That was much less Jean Piaget than it was my Higher Power, just reminding me that I had forgotten about one of the truly great lessons that sobriety and running had in common: *humility.*

Humility takes a lot of forms. And although we may not think so right away, all of those forms are good for us. Running humbles me. Almost every time I run, I am given another lesson in humility. It puts me back in my place, reminding me of my station and general insignificance in the grand scheme of things. And it helps me handle less metaphysical problems. Like coming to terms with being a bigger runner who started running in his late thirties, and understanding how that has a lot to do with why I'm never going to be as fast and effortlessly athletic as someone half my age who weighs 140 pounds and has been running competitively since childhood; it helps with the stark mortification of that first day of truly cold weather when it's time to break out the running tights. Because running is fucking hard, *running humbles me.* Even at the peak of achievement — my fastest 5K, adding an extra ascent of a challenging hill at the end of a hard run, my first half-marathon — it was humility that allowed me to get there. Humility keeps the overreaching excesses of my ego in check; it corrects me when I am out of alignment with who I am supposed to be.

⦿　⦿　⦿

"So, *Stewart*," Stephen said, easing into his chair. "We've never talked about our Scottish names! Are your people Protestants, or micks like mine?" It was my final session with Stephen, and he was relaxed and expansive a few weeks before Christmas, taking the time to delve into our common Scottish heritage.

I told him that my Stewart side descended out of the Quebec woods, a mix of French and Scots. "My apparent Scottish heritage," I explained, "came from my mother's side. She was a Cameron by birth, born in Rutherglen, a suburb of Glasgow, in 1948."

Stephen nodded appreciatively and motioned for me to continue.

"After the war, my grandparents came to Windsor, and the first place they lived was in one of three houses that used to sit on the small peninsula of land at the junction of Wyandotte Street and Walker Road," I said, gesturing through the large office windows, over the bare maples that towered over the neighbourhood, to the plot of land a few blocks east of where we sat, "… where the Tim Hortons is now. But in the 1950s, the three homes fronted on Walker and their backyards met at a point. It was strange, residential plot, nestled in the shadow of the towering Hiram Walker & Sons whisky warehouses and distillery buildings."

Stephen was fascinated. He remembered when there had been a gas station on that plot of land but never knew there had been houses there. "So, they lived there in the shadow of those Hiram Walker & Sons whisky warehouses and distillery buildings?" he asked, referring to the orange-brick buildings that loomed over the intersection to this day, visible out the window above the trees.

"Yeah, and when my mother was a little girl, she would go out into the grassy fields near the warehouses and wait for the distillery workers to come out onto the fire escapes to eat their lunches. And once she had an audience, she would sing to them. They would wrap bits of sandwich and cookies and hardboiled eggs in twists of paper and drop them down to her."

"What a fantastic memory," Stephen smiled. "A red-headed Scottish lass with a big voice. Do you know what songs she sang?"

We talked about the songs — old hymns, show tunes, folk songs; we talked about her being raised in the Salvation Army; we talked about her marriage to my father, which caused tension between my mother's family and the strict Salvationists. As we spoke, I became conscious that through all of this largely unprompted family history I was talking about my mom in the past tense — she *was* a good singer, she *loved* to dance, she *was* a nurse, she *was* a fantastic cook. And although it was the honest and appropriate way to be talking about her, seeing as how she had been dead for eight years by that point, talking about her in the past tense was not something I often did. I became conscious of the fact that Stephen was going to pick up on this detail. And he did.

"She's gone now," he said.

I nodded sadly and told him the tale of the virus that took her life in October 2006, when she was only fifty-eight. "Of all the gifts I have been blessed with in sobriety," I said, "the greatest gift is knowing that when my mother died, she knew I was sober and that the amend I had made was intact."

"That's a very special thing," Stephen said quietly. "I'm sorry she's gone, Robert — *so young!* — but what a gift to be able to give a parent as they leave this life: knowing that their child is happy and healthy ..." A small silence passed. "Well," he said, looking at his watch, "as much as I wish we could sit and talk about our families all day, we should probably talk about why we're here so I can write that letter. Let's talk about the event again. Why don't you take me back to the events leading up to that day in the park?"

Some six months removed from the events in and around the park, I had recounted the story of that day — aloud and in my head — doubtless thousands of times. It had taken on a certain filigreed quality; I felt removed from it, desensitized to its power over me. But apparently, this was all an illusion because at some point in my recitation of Super-Path Saturday, I realized Stephen was down on one knee before me, gripping my shoulders and shouting, "Robert! Robert! Why are you near tears right now! What part of you hurts right now!"

Tears were streaming down my face. A giant sob was caught inside of me. "Right here," I croaked. I pointed at my heart.

"Why does it hurt!" Stephen yelled, his face inches from mine. "*Who did they offend, Robert! Who did they offend!*"

"My mother!" As soon as the answer left my lips, I knew it was the truth.

A huge smile spread across Stephen's face, and he gave me a triumphant shake: "Your mother," he said. "Your memory of your mother, of your parents, your love for them — that's what they offended."

Until that very moment, it had never occurred to me that the reason I punched Chad Poupard in the face, the reason all of this courtroom drama was happening, was because I loved and missed my mother and could not abide someone offending her memory, so very subtly — but very intensely — embodied by Willistead Park. Hell, the whole reason I decided to start running — a story that featured a very portentous walk around the park — began with my failure to make a sickbed promise to my dying mother.

"That was just for you," Stephen said, settling back into his chair, handing me the box of tissues. "I wanted you to have that."

A protracted silence ensued. "How did you do that?" I finally asked.

He knew, he said, that there was some real pain, some greater loss at work; my response that day outside the park was just too visceral to be anything else. I felt such pain that I needed to make it visceral for Chad and Sandra, too. I had inadvertently tipped him off that it was a deeper, familial connection when, in our first meeting, I had, seemingly unconsciously, referred to my mother in the past tense, even though I had not mentioned her death a few moments before while outlining my family history. "I knew I'd excavated an important piece there," he said. "And I wanted to help you see where the excavated piece fit. They offended your mother, and they were going to pay."

If I hadn't been sitting in the armchair across from Stephen when he pulled it off, if I hadn't been the analysand in our tableau, the subject of this therapeutic breakthrough, I likely would have had my doubts about what, on the surface, seems like a very cliché outcome, a punchline right out of a book of Freudian jokes. But he was right. The scenes flicker past the candleflame of memory like the 35 mm negatives of my earliest visits to the park, pulled from a shoebox in the cupboard under the bookcase where the family photo albums were kept in my childhood home on Iroquois Street. My connection to Willistead Park, a public space I've lived within a kilometre of my entire life was elemental: my parents took me for walks there when I was an infant; I played in the park in the fall leaves as a child; it was the locus of teenaged hijinks and high school lunch hours; I walked in it with Jennifer when we were courting; we walked in it with our own children in marriage. I learned to come to this park, to be at home in it, because this is where my parents brought me. And in realizing its connection with my mother, another piece of the puzzle fell into place; I recovered a piece of family history that often flew under the radar, though it was seemingly buried right down in my DNA: My maternal grandmother, Catherine Cameron, and all six of her sisters suffer or suffered from facioscapulohumeral muscular dystrophy (FSHMD) and were all either severely limited in their mobility, or, like my grandmother, wheelchair-bound in the latter years of their lives. As FSHMD is an inherited genetic disorder, my mother was also a carrier, and had she lived past fifty-eight, may have exhibited more symptoms as she aged, though any symptoms that were present were limited to a slight weakening of the muscles in her upper arms as she aged. As preteens in the late 1980s, my sister and I were also tested for FSHMD at Royal Victoria Hospital in London, where we were put through a battery of nerve conduction velocity and electromyogram tests. We were both found to be non-carriers, though the symptoms can manifest out of nowhere, particularly in women, as you age.

It is a strange connection, I realize, connecting my mother so strongly to a public place — a place that is other than home — for this amongst other reasons. But it is no less real for that. Though often forgotten beneath the grief over the loss of my mother and my own return to sanity and health, and the general passing of time, the issue of accessibility was a matter of blood ties, of genetics, of principles, and it had come to the fore. Willistead Park — the values it stood for traditionally, and what it could evolve with the city to represent — loomed large for me, my family, and everyone who cared to enjoy it. Because although many important family moments took place there, Willistead Park was not our private backyard, nor was it ever considered such, and it was all the better and more important for that. By decree of the very people who had bequeathed their homestead to the city in 1921, Willistead Park was *and remains* an open, communal space, a gift from the Walker family to everyone. My mom was all about that kind of generosity. The park was a good place to go to do family things because it was a family place. I wish, to this day, that I was better at carrying out that part of my mother's legacy. I tried to do it in my own way, and I had ended up in jail, in the courts and in counselling. Again.

The truth was as exhilarating as it was cold and stark: Standing there at the intersection of St. Mary's Gate and Niagara Street, before the welcoming gates of Willistead Park on that fine May day, Sandra Voorhees, Chad Poupard, and the rogues' gallery of associated super-path opponents had no idea that they had offended my mother. But they were going to have to pay. And it was going to be an intensely personal statement. There was no grey area here.

Because who had offended my mother more than me? A son who refused to lose weight and live a healthier life in her memory, as per her deathbed wishes. A son who had shrunk at the foot of his mother's deathbed, afraid and too ashamed to look his terminally ill mother in the eye, but not too ashamed to deny her wish, and certainly not afraid to continue eating and gaining weight for another six years after her death.

When I was finally running and losing weight, my biggest regret was that my mother was not there to see what I had done. And I was not anywhere near done feeling guilty and remorseful about that. The gift of the running-shaped hole brought me to this place, to the point of confrontation and crisis, to face the unfinished business with my mother. Anger that I had offended her in her final days spilling over into the park she loved, where I had taken the first overburdened steps on this long, life-altering run. It may not have looked like a story about how running can change your life on the surface, where I logged the endless, sweat-soaked kilometres, but when you got up above the pavement and looked down on it from a heightened perspective, it was clear that running was simultaneously the reason I had something to atone for, and the reason why I was able to atone.

I stood up for my mother's principles when she could not. I was able to stand up for those principles, consequences be damned, because I had fulfilled her wish. I had made good on the deathbed promise I had denied her. And knowing that made all of this a small price to pay.

CHAPTER FOURTEEN

IMMINENT JUSTICE: OR, ROBERT EARL STEWART VS. HER MAJESTY THE QUEEN

THROUGHOUT MY RUNNING career, I had made a point of starting important days with a run, whether what lay ahead was a particularly long and stressful day at work, a long drive to the cottage, my fortieth birthday, or a session in the tattoo parlour. Nothing gets the day off to a good start better than a run — even a bad run. It's invigorating, it boosts confidence, and when I am done running, the hardest part of my day is over. There is nothing I will encounter on a day-to-day basis that is tougher than running.

I shouldn't say *nothing*. Sitting through your first court appearance for assault and mischief charges is, in its intensely staid way, more difficult to endure than a tough run. But even though I had a run scheduled for that morning, I can't account for why I didn't run on the day I appeared before a judge.

Jennifer and I arrived at the Ontario Court of Justice building at 2:00 p.m. to meet up with Johnny Rydel. Jennifer had been holding it together as the court date approached, but as we rode up in the elevator, the worry and fear she had been keeping in check for six months came to the fore and she began to weep silently. When the elevator doors parted, we were confronted with the bustling courtroom-level concourse. She squeezed my hand that much tighter and dabbed at her eyes as Crown lawyers in robes and collars, lawyers of all make and model, myriad clerks, police, bailiffs, and courthouse security bustled about like a scene out of one of my favourite childhood books, *Busy Day, Busy People.* There was also the standard complement of perps right out of Central Casting Windsor lurking in the corners and leaning surreptitiously against the wood-panelled walls, scratching at their track-marked arms and scabrous hands, talking on cellphones, and yelling at their lawyers — all of them under the impression that oversized football jerseys and ball caps with unbent brims and retail stickers still in place were proper court-date attire.

Here was bottom. Not the smack of my knuckles against a man's lips, not the jail cell, not the front porch with my sobbing wife. The realization that in the eyes of the law, in the eyes of my accusers, I was no better — *no different!* — than this rogue's gallery of junkies, pimps, petty criminals, and assorted scofflaws … I felt too warm, too tight about the neck and jaw, numb and fidgety. There had been a terrible mistake. I was a good person. These people had offended my memory of my mother. I was different.

And as the heightened paranoia washed over me in waves, I knew it was a direct result of not having grounded myself in the meditative practice of running that morning. A simple run — even something as brief and unchallenging as a quick, highly symbolic

3 kilometres around the super-paths and back — would have delivered me from these free-floating anxiety blues, replacing them with humility, a sense of well-being, and acceptance. This was real. This was where I was at. This was happening for a reason, and I was going to learn something from it. Knowing that helped tether me back to the moment, but now I was squeezing Jennifer's hand harder than she was squeezing mine.

A small group of friends, including Peter Horvat, who would be called as a character witness on my behalf, were waiting for us outside of Courtroom 10. Johnny Rydel appeared in his barrister's robes and said it was time to go and he ushered us in the officious hush of the courtroom. We slid into a couple of rows toward the back of the room.

When it came time for my case to be heard, Johnny motioned for me to join him at the defendant's table at the front of the room. He had stressed many times that I was not going to jail for this (certainly not today), and that even if the judge determined a trial was necessary — unlikely given my clean record, my plea of guilty, and my anger management work with Stephen — and even if I was found guilty at that ludicrous trial, I would not be whisked off to prison at that time, but would await a sentencing hearing in the comforts of home. Still, as I kissed Jennifer on the cheek, I experienced what I can only describe as free-floating momentousness: equal parts dread, giddiness, indifference — something big was about to happen.

There was some moving of files and shuffling of papers up at the judge's bench during which time I turned in my seat to make eye contact with Jennifer. This was when I saw Sandra Voorhees, in another loud, shapeless floral-print dress, entering the courtroom. She was accompanied by a woman who looked like a younger version of her, one whose vitality had not been destroyed by a lifetime of bitterness and pique. There was still no sign of Chad Poupard, the actual complainant in the matter of assault. The Crown, of course, does not need a victim in the room to continue to prosecute.

The judge, Justice McGregor, called the court to order. Sitting next to Johnny, who exuded calm, I said a quick prayer, asking for the ability to accept whatever was about to happen and vowed never again to skip a run before an important life event.

There were some preliminary boilerplate statements regarding the case number and the like before the justice removed his glasses with an exasperated sigh and leaned forward with his arms folded over the bench. "I'd like to begin by pointing out that this is not the kind of case that typically occupies the court's time," he said, staring directly at the blond-haired Crown attorney, Ms. Grey.

Johnny was sitting back in the chair next to me, one long leg crossed jauntily over the other. He had a smug smile on his face. He seemed to be enjoying himself.

Peering dubiously down at the documents before him, McGregor said, "It is not often a case involving simple assault makes it this far in Superior Court." He returned his glasses to his face and nodded to me, invited me to stand, and asked the clerk registrar to proceed.

The clerk registrar stated for the court that in the case of Robert Earl Stewart vs. Her Majesty the Queen that the accused was being charged on Information Number 141049, an assault on Chad Poupard, contrary to Section 266 of the Criminal Code. She turned to me and said, "To count one, sir, how do you plead, guilty or not guilty?"

"Guilty," I said, for which she thanked me, and Justice McGregor invited me to have a seat next to Johnny.

Standing alone at the prosecution's table, Ms. Grey then ran down the details of the case, careful to drive home the point that I followed my victims to their home, like a stalker. She had clearly bought into the official narrative being pushed by the socialites who made up the core of the Save Willistead Park! crowd — that I had a well-earned reputation as the neighbourhood drunk, the kicker of dogs, the frightener of children, the masher, the degenerate, the bringer of garbage; a man who had waged an extended campaign of terror against a neighbourhood and its good, white denizens. The Crown said she was unwilling to agree to a peace bond because of my extensive (though, I can only assume wholly anecdotal given the lack of a criminal record) background in the aforementioned areas. She was also careful to point out that I was the type of person who thought knocking the cellphone out of someone's hand and punching them in the face was self-defence.

Then it was Johnny's turn to address the court. He had an air of bemusement about him, which seemed to match Justice McGregor's perspective on the entire matter. Johnny clarified for the court that the events of that day were not "all one continuous transaction," that I had retreated to a friend's backyard to get away from Voorhees, Poupard, et al. "The whole issue arose out of some trailways or paving within the Willistead Park area," Johnny said, feigning a detached, blasé, and incomplete knowledge of the trifling matter that had resulted in such a conflagration in the streets. "I didn't know anything about the pathways, but apparently it was a matter of some civic controversy."

The judge didn't care to hear about my returning of the discarded protest signs to Sandra's house. He asked if the assault charge resulted from physical violence pertaining to the pathway matter. Ms. Grey answered that it was.

"A finding of guilt then, on count one," said McGregor. The mischief charge was then withdrawn by the Crown, no longer deemed necessary by my opponent, the Queen, since I'd copped to the more serious offence.

Johnny was then asked to make his submission to the court. In that, he highlighted my education, my work as a journalist, my status as a family man, and my active interest in the Walkerville neighbourhood. He then passed the character reference letters written on my behalf up to the bench — the letters from the various medical doctors, lawyers, members of Parliament, and social justice advocates who considered me their friend and an upstanding member of the community — as well as the letter from Stephen J. Bruce saying I had successfully completed anger management counselling. The judge announced who each letter had been written by, before spending a few silent moments reading each one.

Peter was then called to the stand. Prompted by Johnny, Peter spoke to my contrition in the matter before the court, that I was not a violent man, that I was a published poet, and that Jennifer and I were "strong-willed but sensitive parents" who were raising our children to be readers, "Which is always exciting to see," Peter said, legitimately enthused. "There's nothing more wonderful, I think, than to see a child embrace literature."

When Johnny was satisfied that my effete and gentle nature had been well established, he asked Peter to elaborate on my career as a journalist. Peter rose gamely to the occasion, outlining various awards and community associations my name was associated with as the result of my career in newspapers.

Justice McGregor's eyes flickered between witness, counsel, accused, and Crown.

Johnny and Peter had his attention. "Your Honour," Johnny said, "I'm asking the court to consider an absolute discharge. The Crown's not saying it's contrary to public interest to give him a discharge. They're wanting a conditional discharge. The only thing that would accomplish would be that he would be required to take part in some counselling, which he's done, and that he would be required to keep away from the individual, Mr. Poupard. He's got no reason to go near that person. I don't even know if he knows who that person is, quite frankly, as he is not present in the courtroom today. And he's been on bail, on conditions of release since that time. There's not been any indication whatsoever. So, that's what I'm asking the court to consider. It's just an incident that erupted. He started out that day he was at the park with a picnic, and things escalated."

The Crown outlined the conditions they were recommending: twelve months with conditions to report, any counselling as directed, no weapons, no contact with Chad Poupard or Sandra Voorhees. Ms. Grey stressed the importance of the Crown's wish to have my DNA collected and entered into the international database of criminals, in case I ever decided to take my picnicking shtick on the road, splitting lips and terrorizing gentrified respectability in my wake. "Your Honour's sat in this court long enough to know that a person of Mr. Stewart's socioeconomic and educational background, with potentially influential friends, still find themselves here before the court on matters of a criminal nature," Ms. Grey said. "And although Mr. Stewart's teaching his children to read, I'm sure he's also teaching his children, 'Don't hit,' because hitting is wrong and assault is a crime, and that's why he's here today."

Justice McGregor now turned to me and said, "Anything you want to add, Mr. Stewart?"

If there's one thing sobriety had taught me, it was how to stand up and admit your faults openly and honestly, with nothing but compassion for others, while being ruthless with the self. Thank God I was, and remain, sober.

"Thank you, Your Honour." (I was off to a solid, if not pedestrian, start.) "It's been said a few times that when I left my house that day, I certainly didn't expect that this was going to be the result. We went for a picnic in the park, and I certainly do regret what happened.

"It was a frightening and disturbing afternoon. I ended up in a jail cell when I was supposed to be taking my son to a baseball practice. I ended up sitting on a bench at the cenotaph with a collapsible lawn chair in a bag and remnants of our picnic, waiting to be picked up after being let out of jail, and that was a real low point, to see myself on a downtown street, having been let out the back door of the police station.

"I know I frightened someone that day, and that person's here in the court today," I said, turning to where Sandra sat, glumly, at the back on the far side of the room. "I apologize to them," I said, making direct eye contact with Sandra and dropping my chin in sombre deference to her. "I don't think Mr. Poupard is here today. I physically harmed him, and I regret that.

"It's not something I commonly get involved in, fights in the street, and yes" — and here I looked directly at Ms. Grey, where she sat at the adjacent table, as she was the person who had supplied me with the perfect segue for what I said next — "I certainly *do* take very seriously the raising of my children, and they have no idea that this is even happening in my life. I would not want them to know that this is where I am today. They think we are out Christmas shopping, to tell you the truth. And that's all I have to say, and I thank you."

As I sat back down, I glanced over for Johnny's approval. He looked a bit stunned, and as I moved to ask how I did, he gestured me to silence and just said, "We'll talk about that later," because now Ms. Grey was rising from her seat and addressing the judge.

"Your Honour, Ms. Voorhees's actually here in the courtroom. She didn't approach me or tell me that she was coming, but I see her here now. Mr. Stewart acknowledged that she was here. I think, pursuant to the victim impact statement section of the Criminal Code, that maybe we should afford her an opportunity to say something, if she'd like to, before you pass …"

How the fuck was I the first person to acknowledge that Sandra Voorhees was in the room? I was kicking myself for having acknowledged her, realizing that had I not pointed her out, she wouldn't now be being given the opportunity to totter up to the witness stand and vomit out all of her delusional vitriol.

"So, Ms. Voorhees, this is your opportunity, as often happens in criminal cases, to provide the court with your thoughts and feelings on how this crime affected you, just to briefly outline …" Ms. Grey said, speaking with metered clarity and purpose, as if she were talking to a child. "I usually do this outside of the court," Ms. Grey continued, "but since you're on the stand now, Ms. Voorhees, I'll remind you that you're not here to talk about what you think *should* happen to Mr. Stewart. That's up to His Honour, and we'll talk about that," she said, gesturing to herself and Johnny. "You're here today to describe for the court how you have been affected mentally, emotionally, financially, physically — those kind of things. How has this crime affected you specifically?"

This is where I began to realize that acknowledging Sandra in the courtroom had been a stroke of unwitting genius on *my* part; and calling her to the stand a dreadful, tactical mistake on Ms. Grey's part because the more Sandra Voorhees spoke, the less credible she became.

"Following, I was absolutely terrified, to be honest" she sputtered, choking back great sobs. "I couldn't sleep for a few nights. And what happened was, after it happened, I received some Facebook messages from people saying Mr. Stewart had been saying some nasty things about me on Facebook. We've never even met."

She's not even going to call back to how I tormented her by using the front entrance during her gatekeeping days at the Windsor Star*?!* I was admittedly a bit chafed by her disavowal.

"So, you were fearful, is what you are telling us?" Ms. Grey said, leading Sandra toward the desired narrative.

"I felt that the picnic was a little bit of a thing against me. I think it was a bit of a stakeout. And I think the restraining order should stay," Sandra whimpered petulantly, causing Ms. Grey to all but facepalm herself while Justice McGregor stared at the Crown attorney over the rims of his glasses.

"Just remember, Ms. Voorhees, exactly what you're here to talk about," Ms. Grey reiterated. "How the crime affected you mentally or emotionally."

"I'm just afraid. I'm afraid!" Sandra cried, her face collapsing into melodramatic terror and grief. "I have to close my blinds as soon as it gets dark now. I live on a busy corner. I live on a very visible corner. You can really see my house. You can see into my home if I'm not careful to have my blinds and drapes closed, and it's been a very terrifying experience."

Her implication that I was not above peeking in her windows had Justice McGregor gazing up at the courtroom ceiling.

"All right. I don't have any further questions, Your Honour," said Ms. Grey, beleaguered. "I think she's made it clear to the court where she's at."

Johnny patted my arm, confident but guarded. I turned in my seat and looked back at Jennifer, where she sat surrounded by Peter and a small circle of our friends. She smiled wanly. She was the most nervous person in the courtroom.

Justice McGregor began to speak: "It's not very common for me to have to deal with a situation like this," he reiterated, looking very pointedly toward the Crown. "I see a difference from Ms. Grey's submission in some respects.

"Yes, there are people here," he said, tenting his fingers over the stack of letters on the bench before him, and gesturing into the gallery, "who are good standing members in the community who contribute greatly to the community, and they are friends of Mr. Stewart, and he's called them for a very focused reason, to address this issue on sentencing, but I don't think that puts him in a particular standard that should cause me to be concerned that he's going to be treated differently or better because of that. Ms. Grey has submitted, for example, that he has influential friends, and she has urged me not to lose sight of the fact that we deal with situations like this that typically result in a probation.

"There are some fundamental distinctions, as I see them, Ms. Grey, on that point, and obviously in this case there is no record. He was contrite, as Mr. Horvat indicated, he has taken responsibility, the usual things we are concerned with, and he went to see a counsellor. He has no relationship with these people. It's not like a domestic situation where we're fearful of further contact and we want to restrain that somehow. The eight hundred block of Moy to the eight hundred block of Monmouth — it doesn't make them next door neighbours. They're in the Walkerville area, but they are some distance apart, separated by Willistead Park, as well. The likelihood of them coming into contact together is not very real.

"Ultimately, I am most concerned with the accountability and deterrence in this case, and I think this process that Mr. Stewart has described has been a deterring effect. Being arrested has been a deterring effect; retaining counsel has been a deterring effect; attending here today has been a deterring effect. I don't have reason to believe he's going to reoffend, so I have to ask what benefit would the probation order serve? Would it be for the purpose of counselling to deal with aggressive behaviour? He has no history of aggressive behaviour at all in his past.

"This one day he was agitated by a love for the park and a perspective he had for it, and what Ms. Voorhees had for it may differ, but it is not likely they will come into contact again for that reason, or any other reason at the park, I assume. That issue has been resolved. Those paths have been paved, and that issue is done.

"The counselling, as I said, is not necessary, and it's just totally out of character for him. So, I don't see what the benefit of a probation order would be, other than, as Ms. Voorhees says, to restrain him because she's fearful. As I've indicated, I think this is an out-of-character incident. It's not likely to occur again. Mr. Poupard, wherever he might be, has learned from it. And if for any reason the two should cross paths together, I'm confident nothing more will come of it than that, and they would go on their way.

"So, there are circumstances where an absolute discharge is appropriate, and it is something that's available to me, and it is something that I think Mr. Stewart is entitled to as an appropriate disposition today. So, you will be discharged absolutely, sir. Thank you very much."

And that was it. With a little nod of his head and some shuffling of the papers on the bench before him, Justice McGregor absolved me.

Johnny and I stood, and he pulled me into an embrace. My glasses askew against him, I peered over his arm to where Jennifer, moved to tears, had her hands clasped beneath her chin. I walked through the rail and hugged her for a good long time. In my head, it seems like the entirety of Courtroom 10 was rejoicing. But it was just us. No one else cared. The clerk was already calling out the next case, and we exited, an exuberant lot, into the big bright concourse.

As soon as the elevator doors slid closed, Johnny turned to me: "What you said in there — where'd you learn to do that?"

"I was just being honest, open-minded, and willing," I said. "A little something I picked up in sobriety. It wasn't a practised speech. It's just the way I talk. I meant it."

"Well, it made a big difference. You should consider getting into this line of work. I've got a lot of clients who could learn from you."

○ ○ ○

Funny how quickly everything returned to normal; how quickly I stopped reliving the events of May 31, 2014, in my head, obsessively looping back over details and exchanges, looking for something that could alter the outcome, some little piece of action, of inflection in my voice, that could convince the court that my transgressions, though true, were somehow justified and honourable. I was free of the oppressive weight of criminal charges, a pending trial, and, regardless of how remote, the threat of possible jail time. I was once again running in that place where running is a place, able to step wholly into that running-shaped hole and occupy it and know that, at least for the duration of that particular run, my will was either turned off completely, or harmlessly wholly engaged. It was meditative, it was freeing, and it was normalizing.

Over the next several months, I trained, but I was conscious of my hip and the dangers of overtraining. I was going to live by that old running dictum that going into a big race, it is better to be undertrained, loose, and healthy than it is to be overtrained, stressed out, and injured. When October 2015 rolled around some ten months later, I wouldn't be injured, I wouldn't be facing charges, I wouldn't be a criminal threat to the United States of America — I was going to run the Detroit Free Press Half-Marathon.

o o o

Some four months later, I was out for a run. It was a pleasant spring afternoon. I had just cut through Willistead Park on the running paths and was rounding the corner northbound onto Argyle Road from Niagara (right in front of George Grayson's house) when who did I spot approaching along the sidewalk, pulled along by her two little dogs, but Sandra Voorhees. We drew alongside each other. "Hullo," I said. She turned and looked after me as I ran past, as if she did not know who I was.

CHAPTER FIFTEEN

RUNNING THE LIMBERLOST: CRISIS ON MUSKOKA ROAD 8

AS IMPROBABLE AS it may seem, it was in August 2015 that I learned it is possible for a man to, almost, experience two Gethsemanes.

That summer, when Jennifer, the kids, and I arrived at the cottage on Oxbow Lake, I was unencumbered by legal peccadilloes, more than a year removed from my resignation from the newspaper, writing, and working happily and quietly as a bookseller at Quixotext Bookstore, and, as of New Year's Day, registered to run the Detroit Free Press Half-Marathon. Given my hip injury and my familiarity with the distance, the half seemed like a more rational, attainable, and much less stressful run.

But there was a new problem I brought with me to the Limberlost Forest that summer. Not a hitch in my stride, a hernia, nor plantar fasciitis. No, ever since my absolute discharge, it had become clear to me that I was suffering through some kind of running-based anxiety. Runs that followed only a day or two after invigorating, fulfilling, and confidence-boosting runs were preceded by waves of lingering worry and self-doubt, which became more pronounced when I began training for the half. Worries about chafing, difficult breathing, and injury were definitely part of the repeating repertoire, but a persistent worry about the inability to finish the run, to complete the distance — a fear of failure — was at its core. This performance anxiety could disguise itself as simple fatigue or boredom, or as a sense of being too busy to get out for a run. It had become harder to occupy the running-shaped hole. It was still there. I could feel it. But there was also some resistance there. Rather than obsess about it, I did what I had learned to do in recovery: I let go of the reins and tried to enjoy a more relaxed approach to running. As a result, though, my running was not where I wanted it to be.

Still, I was looking forward to running in the Limberlost. I packed my running gear for the trip, excited at the thought of waking up early and heading out on the roads that ringed Oxbow. I would run, slick with sweat and Deep Woods Off, before returning to the cottage, diving in the lake, and taking up my customary position in a Muskoka chair at the end of the dock with a fresh coffee, my book, and a few handfuls of Picard's Chip Nuts.

My half-marathon training schedule called for me to run 70 kilometres that week. But in deference to family time and going into the Detroit Half slightly undertrained, loose, and healthy, instead of overtrained, stressed-out, and injured, more relaxed runs of 6 to 10 kilometres — maybe 30 kilometres in total — were planned. Also on the loose, Oxbow Lake itinerary was another Krapp Brothers expedition, to make up for the shamefully wanting and embarrassing affair, now three summers past — the aborted adventure to the end of the lake, after which Jennifer snapped that life-altering photo of me at my heaviest, sitting obese and useless in the hull of the canoe.

Setting out from the dock on our third day at the cottage, I sat tall in the stern, wearing a life preserver that was not only rated to support my weight but looked well-proportioned on my frame, allowing me to power our canoe to the stream-crossed copse at the lakehead. Nathanael, Jonah, and Thomasin (yes, our party had grown by one nine-year-old red-headed girl, emboldened to join the team, I would like to think, by her father's vigorous health and physical fitness) were loaded down with their adventure bags stocked with sandwiches, apples, water bottles, and the standard regalia of spies in the Muskokas (notebooks, pencils, magnifying glasses, plastic hunting knives, sunscreen, and bug repellent). We hauled the canoe into the woods, and I showed them how to portage through the bush.

Arriving at the road that had been the welcome impediment to our progress two summers before, we now climbed the embankment with the canoe, braved the open road and charged down the opposite embankment, navigating through a boulder- and deadhead-strewn bog, before setting the hull into Little Oxbow Lake. Small, still, and desolate, the lake had no cottages, no pleasure craft. Just trees hard by the shore all around ... and *a sound*. I instructed the kids to take their paddles from the water, and we floated in silence. From somewhere off to our right on the small, unpopulated lake, muted to a white noise, came the sound of falling water.

A bog backed by a wall of deadfall formed a barrier between us and the source of the sound. Poling our way through dead trees, hummocks of floating turf, and foul mud, we arrived at a waist-deep, rock-lined cistern at the base of a sheer granite face. Cutting down through the granite, we discovered a shaft of light and foam cascading down the crevasse in tiers from some unnamed body of water above.

The Krapp Brothers & Sister did not come this far to turn their backs on such an impressive chasm. Our expedition, our mission, had been fortified by my greatly improved fitness, and by my freedom from irrational fear. We began climbing. Water rushed around our feet and legs as we picked our way up the waterfall, a vertical climb of approximately thirty metres. The chasm, never more than two metres wide, presented our party of brave adventurers a suitable challenge. Finding and calling out foot- and handholds and safe passage to one another, we triumphed, scaling the sheer cliff walls and boulders that had cleaved and tumbled from the walls probably centuries before we had paddled to the foot. The area did not seem well travelled. It was conceivable to think we were the only party to set foot here in recent memory.

At the top, we traced the shallow stream that ran under the forest canopy to the precipice of the chasm to where it rolled in a thin sheet over a partially dismantled beaver dam from another small, desolate lake. That lake, we discovered, almost too late, was carpeted with a deep shag of leeches — one did attach itself to my shin, but I peeled it off and tossed it back into the water with hardly a second thought, much to the kids' astonishment. With the canoe overturned at the lip of the cistern far below, the leeches were our limit. But what a limit it was — the kids hardly believing that such a place existed so close to the cottage, so close to home, even! And I had to agree with them.

We descended the tiers of the waterfall. I took photos; I shot video; we caught and released a fun little frog we found kicking in the cistern. I leapt into waist-deep bog water to haul the canoe back into the open lake. My wide-eyed progeny watched over the gunwales as I broke through water-logged deadfall and bracken, sometimes swimming, sometimes yanking and pushing our way back into the open waters of Little Oxbow, at which time I expertly hoisted myself back into the canoe. We paddled to a large, dome-like rock along the shore of Little Oxbow. We climbed to its summit and sat down to eat our lunch. We composed a letter (the notebook and pencil the boys brought along rising to the occasion) announcing our presence there that day: it stated where we were from, the day on which we arrived at this place, and invited people to contact us via email should they find our note, which we zipped up in an empty sandwich bag and affixed to a tree branch. Included in the map was an Arthur Ransome-esque map of Little Oxbow, with an *X* at the end marking the access to the waterfall, illustrated in by Nathanael.

Jonah fell bum-first into the shallows while getting back into the canoe … but the magic was not ruined. We had made real, lasting memories. We had all seen things we had never seen before. Not only had I been up to the physical challenge, I had been invigorated by it, doing things that two years before would have stopped me short — because of fear and a lack of mobility and cardio capacity and endurance. In the same way my dad had shown me, I had been able to show my children what a father does while at a cottage: lead, instruct, educate, remain calm while a leech attempted to drain my life's blood through my shin … That was all a result of me filling my running-shaped hole.

Upon our triumphant return to the cottage, we spent the rest of the day in the water and at the end of the dock as a family. The sun arced above us, and as the light shifted toward late afternoon, a plan began to form in my head, based squarely in restlessness and that stubborn streak, or mania, that exists in all runners. I'd come a long way — as a person, as a runner, and by minivan! It seemed so pathetically anti-climactic, then, to be back in the Limberlost and to only run a total of 30 kilometres — the distance determined by my half-marathon training schedule — over a seven-day period. It seemed like I was giving myself an out: just saying '*I'm on vacation and I'm relaxing,*' and not pushing myself on the fantasy training terrain I had access to only once a year.

This, I knew, was my disease — my self-consciousness, my fear and self-doubt, my inherent laziness, my fear and boredom, the guilt and shame of the demotivation that had been weighing on me … all of it occluded the place I needed to occupy in order to be sane and happy. The place I could only find running. That day's successful Krapp Brothers mission left me feeling as if I had come of age as a father, and it spurred me on toward coming of age as a runner.

Which brings us to the Gethsemane of 2015. I put down my book and turned to Jennifer: "I feel like I need to run down to the end of Limberlost Road," I said. "And back."

"Right this minute?"

"No. In the morning. I'm going to leave early and run all the way down to the end."

"You can do it," she said. Her support often took this matter-of-fact tone. It wasn't exuberant; it wasn't dramatic. That isn't our style. What it was (and what it remains), was faithful. This same faith had allowed her, even during the worst of my drinking, the worst of my eating, to know that that I was going to get better.

"It's sixteen-point-seven kilometres down to the highway. Then I will come back."

"Well, just bring your CamelBak and your phone," she said. "Don't worry about us."

○ ○ ○

I woke up early and slipped into my running gear. I had filled my CamelBak (a streamlined sports backpack that contains a bladder for liquids — a mouth valve–controlled hose rides over the shoulder so that the wearer can drink from the bladder — that holds three litres of water. I filled the pockets of the CamelBak with a turkey sandwich, a banana, my smartphone. Because that summer was reportedly one of the most active black bear seasons in recent Limberlost memory, I had an air horn and a bear bell tinkling rhythmically in my shorts pocket.

I set out at 9:24 a.m. I was two months out from the Detroit Free Press Half-Marathon, and I had something to prove. Round trip, it would be about 33.9 kilometres from cottage driveway to faceplant in the lake: the longest, most difficult run of my career. I wasn't worried about fluids because I knew I would be able to fill up with water at the public pump at the fire station in the village of Hillside, where Limberlost Road, a.k.a. Muskoka Road 8, meets with Highway 60. However, the smartphone, though an essential long-run supply, was going to be all but useless if I got into trouble. Though I would be able to get a signal once I got out to the end of West Oxbow Lake Road, the chances of Jennifer pulling in a signal, given the cottage's very weak and intermittent cellular coverage, was remote at best.

The air may be cleaner in cottage country, but when the humidity drives the heat up into the thirty-eight to forty degrees Celsius range, no amount of pine forest, Shield rock, and deep cold lake is going to fool your respiratory system into thinking it's hauling good air. Factor in the long, rolling undulations of Limberlost Road, which sometimes climbs upwards of 50 metres drawn out over 2 kilometres, coupled with all the pounding on the hips, buttocks, and lower back on the downward slopes and the fact that the road-cut is wide and well clear of the cooling forest canopy ... It was a tough run.

Despite efforts to let my thoughts play themselves out to a point of silence, I could not get a meditative groove going. I would latch on to scraps of emotion and self-analysis and worry them like beads in the nervous digits of my thinking. In keeping with the pattern of my runs over the past eight months, any confidence I had going in, any uplifting take away from a recent run, slipped away early, carried by a wave of self-doubt. There are some runners who might say this is a good thing; that I was not resting on my self-bestowed laurels; that I was forward-looking and not easily satisfied with past achievements. Such positivity was not present on that day. These thoughts had already colonized my mind as I left the rutted hard-pack and gravel of West Oxbow Lake Road behind and hit the southbound pavement of Limberlost Road. A glance at my watch told me my pace was good given the terrain — about 7:30 per kilometre — but it felt unsustainable, even 4 kilometres into the run. I was already unsatisfied with the end result, and I was nowhere near done.

At around 8 kilometres, I was standing against the guardrail at the mouth of South Limberlost Road, my smartphone in my hand, thinking about ringing Jennifer for a lift. This run was not working for me. Running with a bunch of mental baggage that doesn't dissipate into the ground with each footfall is a very specific variety of Gehenna for this runner.

One of the things that frightens me the most about mental and emotional torment is that it is so fucking boring! No room in the interior life — that precious, heterotopic space — for anything but myopic navel-gazing and rehashed traumas, real or imagined. Where some might thrive on the drama and catharsis, I simply become drained and useless. I can't even decide if I become overstimulated to the point of ennui with my own bullshit, or if the fretting and negativity is totally void of stimulation. Boredom, for me, is not a relentlessly expansive vapidness. It is a frenetic tape loop of calumny: self-important fantasies, rehearsed interior monologues and arguments, and visions of embarrassment and failure. At its best, running *is* an expansive vapidness: a paucity of thoughts with big spaces in between and no apparent theme or thrust. When running is good, it's mindless. When it's bad, it's full of self. And the self, though it can be endlessly fascinating to the self, can also get boring.

I put the phone away in favour of some calf and quad stretches and ran on.

I hit the 12.25-kilometre mark an hour and forty-five minutes out and stopped to eat my sandwich and banana at the foot of a driveway that exited onto Limberlost Road. My thanks to "The Maschmanns" (this according to the wooden sign hanging from the mailbox), who unwittingly provided a soft shoulder to rest on, and a wooden hydro pole, against which I stretched my calves. The food changed my mood a bit. Running all the way to Highway 60 wasn't going to be so bad, and it would easily be landmarked for posterity. But running there would require a somewhat unrealistic return leg. I stood there at the end of the Maschmanns' driveway for a few minutes, wondering if I should make this the turnaround point in a 24.5-kilometre run. Still a massive run, but not what I had set out to do. Maybe this was the run that was going to restore my drive and reinvigorate my passion for running? I owed it to myself — to everyone! — to find out. So, refuelled and rested, I continued south — now at a slight though predominately downhill trajectory — to the highway about 4.45-kilometres distant.

With an eye for a break in traffic, I touched the toe of my running shoe onto the pavement of Highway 60, took a moment to gaze out across Peninsula Lake while sucking on my CamelBak's water hose, and then, before I could unsaddle myself and pull my smartphone out of the bag's side pouch, turned and started back the other way.

A kilometre into the return trip, I realized I was whipped. Limberlost Road reeled out ahead of me, a grey-and-yellow skink through the forest and Shield rock faces. I hadn't stopped running on hills at any point during this entire run. I was either climbing a long, slow incline; thanking my maker that I had reached the brief dome at the crest; making a long, pounding descent; or baking in the breezeless concrete trough in between. Without hangovers to contend with — thank God — the sober runner had to contend with the dreaded Three *H*s: heat, humidity, and hills. I had had to travel 700 kilometres from Windsor and Essex County's unrelenting flatness to experience them, but I had found them here. The experience was immersive.

I was fighting the urge to call Jennifer for a rescue, trying to convince myself that even if I called, the cellular service at the cottage was so bad there was no way she would receive the request. I was either finishing the run, or walking it in. (Or just lying down in a bog until someone came along and found me.)

I was experiencing what it was like to run wholly outside the running-shaped hole. I carried on like this until I ran out of water somewhere around the 22-kilometre mark. It was difficult to believe I'd drained three litres off my back and felt in no way bloated or waterlogged, but my level of perspiration did provide a good explanation for that. What was *really* difficult to believe, however, was that I had forgotten to fill up my CamelBak's water bladder at the Hillside fire station, where ice cold water gushed out of a spigot at the push of a button, metres from where I'd stood at the intersection of Limberlost and 60. Live and learn — or neither.

Tired, hot, and thirsty, my grip on reality was slipping. I was hearing things in the underbrush on either side of the road. I'd silenced my bear bell with the magnetized mesh slipcover that ceases the jingling because it was driving me mad. But that only made it that much easier to hear the dopplering whine of every insect and the crunch and rustle of every small creature of the forest floor. Every time I shoulder-checked, I pretty much expected to find an enraged and abysmally lost grizzly (black bears being both too pedestrian and possibly not even as big as me), or a hill person resplendent in a raiment of human flesh, occult stick sculptures, and animal dung closing the gap on me and my neon orange running shirt. The lack of water became a morbid preoccupation. As did a creeping numbness bordering on absence where I knew my three middle toes should be. (Oddly, this numbness was coupled with a feeling like slivers of glass were being inserted into the oddly disembodied tips of my toes.) No longer obsessing only about water, I was now also confronting the nightmare of taking off my shoes and finding I'd run my toes into aspic.

At some point, I crossed to the east side of the road and just stayed there, with my back to any oncoming traffic. It brought the turnoff to West Oxbow Lake Road closer by mere metres, but in my flagging condition, that was of great comfort. I took a brief walk break, just long enough to send Jennifer a desperate, two-word text: *ride now*. I knew full well that the chances of her receiving it at the cottage were pretty much nil.

The few vehicles that did happen by in either direction contained the standard complement of preppy, young dudes with popped collars at the wheel accompanied by young girls in cut-offs and bikini tops with their bare feet up on the dashboard; or the retirement-aged couple, all L.L. Bean and Tabi International, the matriarch tsk-tsking at the sight of the vagrant shuffling along the gravel shoulder, sucking pathetically on a dry hose that, no doubt they assumed, hooked straight into a wineskin of gut-rotting moonshine or ether. Whether they were judging me or I was judging them, the fact was that it was one of these Audis, Subarus, or Land Rovers that I was going to have to flag down to beg a ride or a sip of their artisanal, distilled well water. I knew that our Dodge Caravan, with Jen at the helm and the kids piled in back, ready with water bottles and fresh fruit and brimming with pride, holding back our Lakeland terrier, Mycroft, who would be wild for a lick at my salty face, would never be the next car coming over the next rise in the road.

A hazy game plan for whatever the end of this run was going to look like was formulating in whatever part of my head was not consumed with staring at my GPS watch as the metres ticked on toward 25 kilometres. The plan was now to hit 29.5 kilometres — the turnoff onto West Oxbow Lake Road. There was no way I would make it up and over its two titanic, unpaved hills. I would arrive at the Canada Post mailboxes for the cottages that ringed that arm of the lake and then I would stop dead and hope someone came and uprooted me.

But the end came sooner than I thought, and the final few metres were nothing exciting. I didn't stop moving when I crossed the 28.5-kilometre threshold because I was afraid I'd lose control of my legs, so I kept walking, eyes on the gravel, hating myself for not being able to make it the final 5 kilometres to the end of the dock. Even though it was my longest, most challenging run ever, I was not happy or proud. I was not full of achievement. The wide-eyed excitement and expectation of the pre-run morning had become the dejected self-loathing of early afternoon. I was disappointed with my effort, disappointed with my time and pace, and disappointed with my inability to handle the hills and the heat. I was livid with myself for mismanaging my hydration so badly, on the verge of tears because I was facing a long walk back to the cottage that included the two very steep West Oxbow Lake Road hills, and I could feel my right foot swelling inside my shoe. I had lost all sense of humility, hubris having completely blinded me to what I *had* achieved.

There was a prolonged lull in the day's occasional traffic.

Then our minivan came into view. My *ride now* transmission had hit its mark. Jennifer had no idea how long it had been since I sent it, but she was sitting in a Muskoka chair on the dock when her phone (at her side primarily for use as a camera while the kids frolicked in the lake), beeped during a rare and fleeting window of cellular reception. I'd only been walking for about twelve minutes when she found me. I made a final crossing to the west side of Limberlost Road, heaved myself into the van, and faked being happy with myself for my darling wife and kids, who were awestruck with my run.

"Where else did you go, Papa?" asked Thomasin. "Like, you weren't running that whole time you were gone."

The boys were laughing.

"Yes, honey. I ran all the way down to the end of the road, and then —"

"And then you ran all the way back to here?!" She pulled an incredulous face.

Mycroft came leaping into my lap from the back seats and began licking my salted neck and face (much to everyone's delight), saving me from having to say something positive about my run.

Jennifer filled in the blank better than I would have: "Isn't Daddy amazing, honey? That's even a long drive in the van!"

"I hope you were safe, Papa," she said. "What if a bear came after you!"

I rang my bear bell, and she was satisfied that I had conquered the Limberlost in safety.

○ ○ ○

The rest of that Sunday is a wash. I remember crawling around like a man-child in the shallows off the dock. I remember an inability to get comfortable in a Muskoka chair. I remember collapsing on the bed. I remember waking up hours later. I ate about a dozen s'mores at the campfire that night and fell asleep in my camp chair before the flames.

When I woke up the next morning, I was in bed in the cottage. Everyone else was already up. It was near lunch. My body ached. I was still angry at myself for falling short of my goal even though I'd run farther than ever before, and now I could add overeating to the list of things I could whip myself for.

The s'mores orgy was symptomatic of a very real problem I'd read about in a few running magazines and heard from some more experienced runners: it's not uncommon for runners training for marathons to actually gain weight, despite the marathon training program's ramp-up in weekly mileage. Since beginning my training program in June, some two months before, I'd put on about twenty pounds. It was a terrible secret. I could see it — on the scale, in photos, in the fit of my clothing — and I just hoped other people couldn't. My body was burning through a ton of calories, and I was ravenously hungry — a tragic by-product of training if you happen to be a bigger runner who has crazy overeating issues.

Oxbow Lake was my favourite place in the world, but I was not in a good place. I was in a slump with my training; I was stressed out and cognizant of depression stalking the edges of everything, and I was terrified of being ill-prepared for Detroit.

o   o   o

Running had been such a new and freeing thing in the summer of 2013. But by the summer of 2015, I had expectations for and about my running, which meant my expectations for myself were exorbitant, and a rigorous training schedule that, with the addition of my 28.5-kilometre run two days previous, was going to make one week at Oxbow Lake tougher than any job I'd ever had. This went squarely against my oft-cited vacation criteria that *no vacation should ever be more difficult than my job*. But running was not my job. Running was supposed to be joyful and glorious and restorative.

It was a quiet, rainy Oxbow Lake morning. I was out in nature, doing something I hadn't been able to do (nor dream of doing) three years before, running along a road I have never been on before ... Why, then, was I thinking about how much I hated running? About how very badly I wanted to get back to the cottage, pull up my familiar spot on the couch next to the wood-burning stove, pick up the novel I was reading, and let the stormy afternoon slip on by? It was not lost on me that when I left the cynical, deadline-driven world of the professional journalist for the comparatively less stressful world of indie bookstore management and bookselling, there had been a corresponding decrease in my passion and commitment to running.

This was what was going on in my head as I ran north along Limberlost Road, up around the bend past Olympia Sports Camp, two days after the toughest run and the greatest achievement to date in my running life. There was thunder in the distance; a rookery of large ravens landed on the road ahead; rainwater was dripping through the trees and down to the forest floor on both sides. It was like something out of a movie: a little bit frightening and danger-ous; totally cool and exhilarating. Better yet, it was like that feeling I used to get when I found myself quite literally in a poem, whether I was standing atop a conservation-area hawk tower or pushing a cart through the grocery store. I would be suddenly scrambling for my pen and notebook, wondering how long the poem had been go-ing on around me. Had I missed a bunch of important stuff, or had I clued in right away? Not just mental, the onset of a poem used to be a full body experience: my ears piqued, my breath became shal-low. The heart slowed; the mind tried to wrangle the full payload of possible thoughts and judgments to the point where it was as open and fertile as a raw wound in the earth; the pupils, I'm sure, dilated for maximum inpouring of raw materials ... I felt I was on the precipice of all of this, some kind of creative bleeding edge, some new synthesis of the running-shaped hole. But the precipice was as far as I would get.

It had become clear that if I was going to have continued success as a runner, I was going to have to accept what many more experi-enced runners had told me repeatedly: *Sometimes you're not going to like running.* So, I stopped feeling as if I had to always be giving off positive vibes about running. Running did not come with some kind of talismanic guarantee of mental health. It was okay to be struggling. I didn't have to feel like I was somehow a fraud because

I was having a hard time staying motivated. That didn't mean I stopped running. If anything, accepting how I felt about my lack of enthusiasm for running and the associated weight gain allowed me to relax and be more realistic about my running. Fear and embarrassment were not going to push me through to the Detroit Half, but the honesty and humility I found in realism would.

That being said, I'd be damned if I would let self-consciousness, anxiety, and fear make me miss my third consecutive Detroit Free Press race.

CHAPTER SIXTEEN

DOUBLE-BOOKED

THREE-AND-A-HALF weeks prior to the half-marathon, I was standing behind the sales counter at Quixotext Bookstore sipping a coffee when the store owner, Mal Peters, popped his head out of the press offices and said, "Where are we with BookFest?"

This struck me as kind of a strange non-sequitur on a fall afternoon. I had known the festival was coming up in a few weeks, but I wasn't too keen on going: the festival lineup had left me a bit flat and, more importantly, that weekend was Detroit Free Press Marathon weekend. I planned on taking it easy leading into that weekend, before being extremely busy for a couple of hours on the Sunday morning. So, I replied in the most blasé and non-committal way I could: "Oh, I might stop in for a bit on the Saturday," I said. "Maybe check out the poetry salon. You?"

Mal was completely unfazed: "No, I mean as far as book orders and organization. Have you been in touch with the committee? Have they given you a full list of attending authors?"

"Oh, that," I lied, feigning nonchalance. "Not yet. I'll email her again right now."

That satisfied Mal, and he disappeared back into the press offices. Of course, I hadn't exchanged word one with anyone on the BookFest Windsor committee because, until about twenty seconds prior, I had no idea I needed to. Apparently, several months before it had been decided by the festival committee and Mal that Quixotext would be the exclusive on-site BookFest Windsor vendor, but no one had bothered to tell me. We were three weeks out from festival kick-off, and I was just learning how my time and efforts had been pledged to setting up, stocking, organizing, and staffing an off-site bookstore over a four-day literary festival. On the fourth day of the festival there was a big Sunday brunch event — something called a Bootlegger's Brunch — at the posh Hiram Walker & Sons Reception Centre on Riverside Drive. This coincided exactly with the morning of the Detroit Free Press Half-Marathon.

Strange, but the part-time job I had taken on as a means of affording me the time to finish the book I was writing about running had become a full-time job that had taken away nearly all of my writing time, impinged on my running schedule, and was now creating a stress load that was, without question, going to be a major distraction going into race weekend.

For the three weeks leading up to the festival, I was logging upwards of seventy hours per week in the bookstore. Over fifty thousand dollars in event stock was ordered, received, and stored. A BookFest staff was cobbled together out of Quixotext Press staff, friends, and my children. Somehow, everything got done. And somewhere in there I managed to bust off a 22-kilometre training run that took me west along the riverfront and along County Road 20, deep into LaSalle, culminating with a triumphant charge up the standard-issue Essex Region Conservation Authority hawk tower at the Petite Côte Marsh. Maybe what I needed to keep my interest in running piqued was some adversity, something to run against? Something that made the running-shaped hole a necessary retreat, a refuge?

o   o   o

On the Friday of BookFest, two days before the half-marathon, I snuck away stateside to another festival: the Detroit Marathon Health & Fitness Expo. Attending the Expo was even more compulsory than my attendance at BookFest. Because the Expo served as the race kit pickup locale for all runners, and because the Marathon and International Half-Marathon and Marathon Relay include two border crossings, showing up in person, passport in hand, to pick up your race kit and your race bib, was *mandatory*. If you didn't do it, you didn't run.

I arrived at the Cobo Center at around 1:40 p.m. and got in line. The line snaked through the expansive concourse for what must have been a kilometre. Once the double set of steel doors that led onto the convention hall floor opened, the actual receiving of the race kits at the long bank of tables that took up a fractional strip of the floor space took all of two minutes.

Race kit in hand, I was only too pleased to spend part of the afternoon wandering the Health & Fitness Expo that took up the rest of the cavernous hall, and whose maze-like aisles comprised the only pathway out. As one of the event's primary sponsors, New Balance, my running gear purveyor of choice, had a full-scale shoe store on-site. Two young, lithe, smiling attendants worked the kiosk. I wandered over to see if, per chance, there was any update pending for my trusty 1340V2s, and somehow, I nearly walked away in a brand new, steeply discounted pair of 860V5s. At one point, I had them on my feet and, despite my knowing that they weren't nearly enough shoe for me — not posted heavily enough, not broad enough through the midfoot, not rigid enough to control my overpronation (excessive inward rolling of the foot) — I even heard myself telling the young fellow who laced them up for me that I was actually going to buy them. That's when I realized that these two young, attractive salesfolk weren't the newbies who'd drawn the short straw and were seconded to the Detroit Expo mobile sales team but, rather, two highly effective New Balance gunslingers, parachuted in to sell new running shoes to people who, though they often obsessed about their shoes, were forty-eight hours out from the start of their race, and likely not looking for a new pair to break in.

"So, which race are you running?" the chipper young salesgirl asked as she knelt before me, measuring up my feet with her Brannock Device.

"Oh, just the half," I demurred.

She bolted up and met my gaze. "'Just the half'!? Like hell 'just the half'!" she said. "You mean 'the motherfucking' half!'"

She was right. I was being too modest, cutting myself down to size before the race had even started. I was guilty of dismissing her as just another pretty girl; now I could see that she was a ninja-level sales associate.

"You're right," I said. "I shouldn't say it like that."

"Listen," said her male counterpart, taking a knee before me and placing both hands on my shoulders, "You are the athlete on Sunday. Thousands of people are going to line the streets in two countries to cheer you on. They don't stop cheering once the elites have gone by. They keep cheering. They cheer louder when the people who are just like them go by."

"Louder," the young lady emphasized.

"So, you be proud, brother. Run *proud*. You worked for this. It's not '*just*' an anything. This is your race. Run hard, but man — have some fun!"

For a few moments it was as if we, in our little huddled trium-virate, were the only three people in the giant Expo centre. I kind of felt bad about not buying the shoes.

o o o

My trip to pick up my race kit also allowed me to play cross-border courier for the day. BookFest Windsor presented the bookstore with the perfect venue for unveiling the new Quixotext tote bags. One hundred of the bags were waiting for pickup at a screen-printing outfit tucked away in Detroit's Eastern Market district. The trans-action took all of two minutes. The box of tote bags in the van, I was on my way back to the border.

I was going to simply pay the border toll on the U.S. side on the way home. They're usually happy to see the back of you, and they don't care what you're carrying out of the country. I'd been told by co-workers there was some additional processing of forms that had to be done in one of the Customs building on the Canadian side, but first I had to pass through Customs.

The Customs booth window slid open, and I handed my passport and the paperwork for the one hundred tote bags to the Canadian Border Services agent — this one a large, middle-aged fellow with the obligatory, quasi-military moustache. He looked at the paperwork, looked at me, and said, "What the hell is this sup-posed to be?"

"It's the paperwork for one hundred screen-printed tote bags I picked up at a screen printer's in Detroit," I said, knowing full well that that is exactly what it said on the very standard and parochially common Canada Customs import forms that had been filled out to exacting CBSA online specifications before I had left bookstore that morning. "The totes are in a box in the back," I said, gesturing helpfully over my shoulder.

"But this isn't filled out correctly," he said, already at full bluster. "Who filled these out?"

"They were filled out by people I work with," I said. "I realize there may be some additional paperwork that needs to be completed inside."

"Yeah, but who sent you here? Who filled out this paperwork?"

"People I work with."

"And where do you work?"

"Quixotext? A bookstore just a few blocks down Wyandotte here —"

"So, they just hand you some papers and you drive into the United States and bring stuff back into Canada? How well do you know these people? How often do you do this?"

"Well, this is the first time — look, if there's something that has to be filled out, that's why I came to see you. This is not a regular part of my job. I just happened to be crossing the border today on a non-work-related matter, and I said I could stop off at the screen-printing place, pick up the tote bags, and bring them back. They filled out the paperwork online and said the person at the border would tell me what to do."

"Do you realize," he growled, eyes bulging, face turgid with his out-of-control systolic, "that I could give you a two-thousand-dollar fine and have you thrown in jail right here and now for not having this paperwork filled out?"

I felt my half-marathon slipping away with each volley of this exchange. The border could either be extremely porous, or intractably dense, depending on your attitude and the whim of the Customs agents on both sides. One false note, one quip or barb could turn you into a "non-desirable" or "enemy combatant" with a single mouse click. "Barred from entry into the United States" was no way to go into race weekend, especially with the start and finish line lying on the American side of the river. Everything I had talked about in my anger management sessions with Stephen, and things I had learned talking with sober friends and advisers played quickly on the tapes in my head. To no avail.

"I believe you about the fine," I said. "But as far as the throwing me in jail part goes, I think you're absolutely full of shit."

His stool shuddered audibly beneath him. "Full of — what?! Full of ... Listen, we can go all night here. This is a federal offence. I can deny you entry to Canada and deport you to the United States, and then they send you back here, and then I send you back to them, saying you've been denied entry —"

"Yeah, yeah, Border Roulette. Heard of it. If there's some additional paperwork that needs to be filled out, I'd like to get it taken care of." I was having too much fun watching him grind his teeth and puff up his Kevlar-encased bulk.

"What's this outfit you work for called again," he asked, desperately trying to control his rage while clicking his standard-issue CBSA pen furiously over a clipboard.

"Quixotext. Just like it sounds. And while you're writing that down, what's the name of the outfit you work for?"

"Son, I *do not* work for an *outfit*," he barked, leaning out his window and as close to my face as his Kevlar body armour would allow. "I work for the Government of Canada."

"Yeah, I know. And you're doing a shit-poor job representing them today," I said.

He folded my paperwork up, handed it to me curtly, and said, softly, "Okay, that's how it's going to be."

"It has been so far, yes."

"You can go right on in there and deal with them," he said, indicating the CBSA Commercial Imports Custom House. He picked up the phone receiver hanging on the wall of his booth and smiled as I drove away.

I sat in the van for a moment when I pulled up in front of the Customs house. Who did he call? He didn't call his wife to have her heat up the meatloaf. Should I just shove my race kit in the nearest trash receptacle? I said a quick prayer, then walked blithely through the automatic doors. A young woman in a CBSA uniform was sitting at the counter behind bulletproof glass. She smiled as I slid my paperwork through the stainless-steel trough.

"I'm bringing in one hundred tote bags. I just have to finish filling out the forms," I said, nodding toward the baskets of barcoded stickers that sat on a series of desks lined up against the wall a few feet away. I knew they had something to do with why I was there and wanted to impress upon this bookish, doe-eyed lass that I was, if nothing else, an old hand at importing small quantities of silk-screened canvas tote bags across the border.

"Oh, no problem," she said. "Yeah, you just need to go over there and put one of those barcode stickers at the top of each form —"

My papers were snatched out of her hands by a woman whose dark hair was pulled back in a bun so tight that a thumbnail drawn gently across the hairline would have likely peeled her scalp off in a rolling flap. She was wearing what can only be described as full CBSA regalia. I swear there were epaulets, scrambled eggs, braided cords, and fruit salad all the fuck over the front of her uniform.

"How come these aren't filled out properly?" she snapped.

"Because I just got here, and I was just about to —" I changed tacks. I was dealing with border brass, apparently. "Am I in the right place? Did I do something wrong?"

"Yes, you didn't finish filling out your paperwork," she snapped. The doe-eyed lass stared at her monitor, afraid to make eye contact with me or her superior. "We could fine you fifteen hundred —"

I changed tacks again. Half-marathon be damned. "Is that all?" I asked. "That guy out there in the booth told me it was two grand. Sounds like somebody might be pocketing a bit of graft off the top —"

"Why would you try to cross the border without your paperwork completed?"

"I came to you, under direction of your co-workers, to complete these forms by putting those barcoded stickers over there on each one of these pieces of paper. If the only place in the world I can get the proper barcoded stickers to complete these forms is right here in this room, and everything I've done right up to walking through these doors and handing this young lady my paperwork is absolutely standard procedure … why is everyone acting as if this is the most unorthodox and inappropriate border crossing they've ever seen?"

"I don't think anyone is acting like that," she sniffed. She handed my paperwork back through the bulletproof glass and stalked off.

Three rectangular stickers, about three inches long apiece, placed unceremoniously across the top of each form. That's all it took. I did it all by myself. I handed the papers back through the trough under the bulletproof glass. The barcodes were scanned. The mouse was clicked. A few keystrokes later and I was back out in the parking lot, just off the corner of Wyandotte and Goyeau, free to go. No one had even looked at the tote bags.

And from the moment I left the Customs plaza until the moment I was safely through the U.S. Customs on race day, I would be envisioning that irate Customs agent smile at me as he picked up the phone receiver in his booth, hopefully not flagging our minivan for some Free Press Marathon morning Border Roulette.

○ ○ ○

When Saturday night's BookFest readings ended, it was time to pack up the entire festival bookstore and vacate the Capitol Theatre. A select few hundred of the books had to be moved to the brunch event venue for Sunday morning. I would be done running the half when the brunch began, but there was no brunch buffet majestic enough to make me show up. I'd arranged for two Quixotext colleagues to work the Sunday morning, and I'd recruited an additional four Quixotext staffers to help with the teardown/relocation effort. But, before we had even boxed a single book, one of the press-office publicists approached and said, "Yeah, we're all going to split. Mal invited us to go out drinking with some of the authors."

I looked in the direction of his slight nod to where Mal Peters stood, smiling smugly while partially obscured by a potted palm.

I'd wanted to be in bed by 10:00 p.m. I had to run 21.1 kilometres in the morning. I'd planned on begging off any heavy lifting, limiting my involvement to directing traffic — hell, I'd originally planned to spend the two days leading up to the half-marathon in my pyjamas, staying loose and relaxed … but instead, I'd coordinated the entire book-sales aspect of a literary festival and ended off the night carrying several hundred boxes, many of them weighing upwards of forty pounds, up and down a staircase, out into a cold fall rain, packing them into my van, then driving everything back to the bookstore, hand-bombing it all back into storage in the office, doing the day's cash-out … It was after midnight — less than three hours before the alarm clock ripped the entire family, all five of us, into consciousness — when I collapsed into bed.

CHAPTER SEVENTEEN

THE FULL HALF

Talmer Bank Detroit Free Press Half-Marathon
Sunday, October 18, 2015

TWENTY-SEVEN THOUSAND OF us faced west along Fort Street, looking up as one from our corrals at the bottom of the Art Deco canyon as snow began to fall out of the dark-purple pre-dawn sky of an October Sunday. It wasn't a lot; it might barely have qualified as flurries, but an audible gasp rose from our mouths as the anxiety and anticipation of the start was momentarily undercut by this cinematic moment.

And just as faintly as it had started, it stopped.

There were probably those for whom the snow, as light and fleeting as it was, meant they were woefully under-dressed or well outside of their familiar climatic zone. But for me — in that moment of reprieve when everyone's face turned skyward as if to catch a flake on their tongue — I knew I was ready and in the right place. It is hard to be full of fear, self-doubt, and uncertainty when you're standing with a bunch of strangers in the downtown core of America's most down-and-out and dangerous city when it looks, for just a few seconds, like you're all there for some grand-scale holiday magic Sears commercial.

Then the horn went off. The part of me used to running local 5Ks capped at five hundred runners wanted to surge forward. But, as I was not one of North America's elite runners, I had to wait, stationed as I was at the back of Start Corral L.

Some twenty-two minutes after the initial sound of the horn, Corral L crossed the line and I was off on a 21.1K international adventure, a run that for the past two years had eluded me as a result of, variously, circumstance, injury, and criminal charges.

I almost didn't care what happened this third time, as long as I started. Finishing would just be a bonus.

○   ○   ○

I knew how excited the kids were on race day because when the alarm sounded at 3:00 a.m. they were out of bed before I was. They were sitting in the living room, in winter coats, boots, toques, and gloves when I descended. They had logistical questions:

"Are we dropping you off and then coming home and then going back to pick you up?" asked Jonah (who apparently had missed several family conversations over the past week about how race day was going to play out).

Nathanael was disgusted with his younger brother "Jonah, that doesn't even make sense — will there be food there?"

Jonah's eyes lit up: "Yeah! Will they have baloney buns or anything like that?"

Thomasin was more focused: "Did you poop, Papa? You don't want to be out there running and have it — you know ..." And here she shook her backside and gestured to what it would look like if poop fell out of a person's bum and ran down their leg to the ground. It was funny enough to make her brother forget about food.

Armed with small brass safety pins, Jennifer and the kids took turns fastening the corners of bib No. 16772 to the front of the shirt I would be running in, and then I donned a selection of clothes that had been tight on me at 368 pounds.

There's a tradition in big city, cold-weather races to wear warm clothes to the starting corrals, clothes that you can discard on the street when the gun goes off. The clothes are then collected by race volunteers and distributed to the homeless. My outfit was comprised of a pair of dark-grey windbreaker pants that ballooned clownishly around my legs, and a XXXXXL shirt in a hapless shade of cranberry. The outfit, though warm in the pre-dawn chill, was a humbling (and frightening) reminder of where I'd been.

Of course, as we neared the border, I began to wonder what the Homeland Security officers on the American side of the Windsor-Detroit Tunnel would make of the man wearing the enormously ill-fitting clothes sitting in the front passenger seat, his pockets stuffed with coffee-flavoured energy gels and a plastic tube of anti-chafing protection. Also, how would the tenor of their opinions regarding my outfit change when they were pulling me out of the van, in front of a stunned Jennifer and the kids, because the licence plate and my passport had been red-flagged by my new CBSA friends following Friday's tote-importing fiasco — a possibility I had failed to mention to Jennifer, or to anyone else, for fear that saying it aloud would only make it more likely to come to pass.

It was just after 5:00 a.m. Surprisingly, the Customs plaza on the Detroit side was not as busy as I'd expected it to be two hours before the race start. We pulled up to the Customs booth. The Homeland Security agent took our passports and the children's birth certificates and asked where we were headed. He asked if I was running the half or the full and seemed satisfied when I said, "the half." And with this we were allowed to pass into the United States. I took it as a sign that I was meant to run this race on this day.

We parked in an underground municipal lot accessible off Jefferson Boulevard and walked as a family to the Cobo Center. Runners give off a strange energy before a race — part anxiety/ dread, part intensity/competitiveness — and it was filling the Cobo Center like a protean sublimation. Not liquid, not solid, not gas, it was just a powerful vibe that, if you are anything like me, is just going to annoy you unless you find people who are on exactly your wavelength.

The Cobo Center concourse — the same place I'd stood in line waiting for the race kit pickup and Health & Fitness Expo two days before — was well lit and filling up. The early morning city was coming into view hard against the eastern exposure's glass wall. People were stretching, doing full-on calisthenics on the hypnotically florid carpeting, eating and lounging on the cavernous concourse's many conversationally arranged couches and chairs, exchanging stories of past road racing triumphs and disasters. Their various entourages (you could always tell who comprised the entourage based on who wasn't wearing running gear and was not talking about running), were, like my entourage, bulked up in winter coats and carrying bags of running gear and race supplies. We found a place at the base of a pillar, along the western edge of the concourse, far enough away from others so as not to be bothered by their conversations.

I was nervous. Scared, even. This was a huge event, and the psychic tension and emotional charge of this huge room and the downtown core surrounding it were making me edgy.

I forced myself to sit down against the pillar, whipped down my oversized windbreaker pants, and not concerned about who saw that part of my body where the leg meets what is technically the groin, applied Body Glide to the region (my plan being to build up layers of viscosity and protection over the next hour or so). Then I decided I would check out the line for the men's room.

While a forced and drunken jocularity is typical of the lines for the *pissoir* at sporting events, this line was a rather grim, silent affair. There was none of the locker-room humour one would expect from one hundred men waiting to relieve their bladders. There really wasn't even any talk of running, which seemed almost impossible, given there were hundreds of runners standing in a line. No matter. I was distracted by the act of waiting for something other than the starting line.

When I crossed the threshold into the washroom itself, I realized why the silence was so pervasive. Unlike those in the liquor-soaked lines at Comerica Park or Joe Louis Arena, the comrades in this line were people who were not so much looking to relieve their bladders as they were hoping to void their nervous bowels. The smell was pervasive. The sound was … also pervasive. And now the reason why the line had been moving so slowly also made sense: everyone was waiting for the stalls, of which there were five. There was almost always one of the three urinals going unused.

It was interesting to see the look of miffed indignation pass over the face of each bladder-holding runner who, once he had stepped into the tiled fluorescence of the washroom itself (and once he had recovered from the head-snapping bitterness resulting from a solid hour of bowels being emptied in splashing, acrid, grunting torrents), realized that his time in the line could have been cut by several minutes had word been sent out from the door and back down the line to let those waiting only to urinate know there was a least one urinal free. Knowing that I was essentially advocating for the creation of a second, special class of bathroom queuing, I heard myself calling this out to the room, over the spackling of porcelain that went on uninhibited and without end behind the closed doors of the stalls, there was generally agreeable muttering in return.

Bladder emptied, I returned to where Jennifer and the kids were holding down our plot around the pillar. The kids had recently annexed a couch and had just finished several scintillating rounds of a game they were calling Hide the Mittens.

"I can't sit still," I said. "Do they need a fourth?"

"I would just leave them alone" said Jennifer quietly. "So far, no one has asked about food."

I asked her for the bagel she had packed for me in her purse. With about forty-five minutes to go before the start, I wanted to have some calories queueing up in my system. As soon as I ate the bagel, though, the breakfast I had eaten at home made it known that it was ready to exit.

Not thrilled with the grim prospect of getting back in line for the washroom, the thought crossed my mind that maybe I could just hold it. Of course, I didn't want to risk soiling myself on an I-75 off-ramp at the 17-kilometre mark. Nor did I want to nearly die of a bowel obstruction at the finish line. So, back to the back of the line for the men's room I went, grimly waiting my turn to plant my taut runner's haunches on an institutional toilet seat well-warmed by the buttocks of hundreds of other runners.

I actually made eye contact, despite all intentions not to, with the gent who preceded me in the stall closest to the washroom door. It was enough to throw lesser men off their race plans, but this was no time for modesty or concerns that the layers of Body Glide I had applied to my inner thighs (I now saw prematurely) were going to act as a waxy adhesive for all that remained on the seat from those who had gone before. I stepped into the stall as the roar of the previous gent's flushing echoed around me. I was relieved to see the bowl was clean, the rim equally so (though I gave it a quick wipe-down), and that there was ample stock of toilet paper.

Gastrointestinally prepped and as self-satisfied as a potty-training toddler after his first successful on-point poop, I strode up to Jen and the kids in the rapidly filling Cobo Center concourse and announced that I was ready to go to the starting line.

Ten minutes and a few blocks southeast later, I emerged from my XXXXXL cocoon, ditched my old clothes in the gutter, and after hugging Jennifer and the kids, I slipped through a gap in the steel crowd-control barrier and stepped out onto Fort Street amidst my 2:35 goal time brethren in Corral L.

●　　●　　●

I was westbound on Fort Street, surprised at how quickly downtown Detroit gave way to what could easily be mistaken for the industrial edge of town. Detroit Police patrol cars and sawhorse barriers blocked every intersecting side street. Foot patrol, mounted police, race officials, and medics lined the route: a mix of alleyways, service shops, greasy spoons, midcentury municipal infrastructure, light manufacturing, abandoned lots, and boarded up storefronts. And they were joined, even at this early hour, along this blighted commercial stretch of Fort Street, by Detroiters: out in force, shouting encouragement, holding up signs, clapping, chanting, singing, and creating a clamour with cowbells.

In the time in took me to clear downtown Detroit, the sun had come up. Ahead, arched across the morning, the span, struts, and suspension cables of the Ambassador Bridge — the phase of the race everyone frets about while telling you how beautiful it is to be crossing just as the sun rises from under the limn of Essex County. I realized the little motes of movement I saw on the traffic-stilled international span were runners southbound into Canada. (Yes, *southbound*. The Windsor-Detroit border being that anomalous spot where commonly held beliefs about north and south in relation to Canada and the United States are delightfully inverted.) And though I hadn't been able to experience the powerful, cinematic moment of the sunrise from the deck of the bridge, like a scene from the symphonic "O Canada" montage they used to screen in theatres before the movies — breathtaking, inspiring, nearly tear-inducing in its grandeur and majesty — I was glad that other runners had.

At the 1.5-kilometre mark at Fort Street and Rosa Parks Drive, I was about eleven minutes into the run. It seemed impossible that there were already runners in another country. Even taking the staggered corral start times into consideration, this seemed super-human. But rather than make me feel small, slow, and alone, this realization did that thing that running always does to me in spite of my diseased nature: it took me so deep it got me out of my self; by separating me from self at depth, it made me feel part of. There were some runners who got to see that sunrise from the deck of the bridge, and I was following the trail they blazed.

A quick glance back over my shoulder into a bobbing sea of faces and bright running gear extending back into the mouth of downtown's canyon and I knew that I was nothing more than a moving point on a continuum of athletes of all shapes, ages, and sizes. Every single one of us was working to complete a goal that had different time signatures, but that goal had the same coordinates; every single one of us was dealing with some flavour of fear, some variant of apprehension, some personal demon that either urges us to stop running, or will never be satisfied, no matter how far we go. It put me at ease. It helped me settle into the seven-minute-per-kilometre pace that I would hold for the next two and a half hours.

By the time you're on the Ambassador Bridge, you've already run on a good kilometre's worth of on-ramp in the bat-shit crazy Customs plaza on the U.S. side, created using the "Let's see how many switchbacks we can cram into this fucker" design principle. It was somewhere in the mindless spiralling and backtracking beneath bridge-owner Matty Moroun's government-terminated second span — it mirrors the trajectory of the original bridge but stops in mid-air before it even gets out over water — that I watched as a runner was stopped and surrounded by a Homeland Security foot patrol. They were shouting at him, "Where's your race bib?! You have to have a race bib!" and he was gesturing back toward downtown Detroit. In the few seconds it took me to pass by the scene, his plight became clear. Overheating in his bulky warm-up wear during the early part of the run, he had discarded the article of clothing on which his race bib was pinned and continued on his feckless way.

It is a well-known feature of every organized race, from the lowliest charity 5K to the most prestigious marathons in the world, that a participating runner must have their race bib pinned and visible on the front of their body. It's stated in your registration. It's part of the race FAQ. So, the fact that he wasn't wearing one was a problem.

I could hear one of the Homeland Security agents yelling into a walkie-talkie, giving the runner's name to a race official somewhere, probably so it could be cross-referenced with the man's name, age, home address, etc., and part of me thought, *Hey, at least they're trying to help this guy out and not fuck up his time too badly.* But another part of me — the part of me that obsesses about tragedy and large-scale news events — was uncomfortable with all of this going down at the foot of the Ambassador Bridge: the world's busiest international border crossing, the conduit for 50 percent of Canada's economy, and widely publicized as the No. 1 terrorist target in Canada.

Yes, aside from proving you're not a bandit — that you've paid to run the race — the race bibs are also used to track runners along the course and act as a stand-in for your passport, which had to be presented, have its number recorded, in order to receive your race

kit. I would loathe to have this guy allowed — through the ubiquitous and officially unexplained "relaxing of security measures" that
precede nearly all assassinations and terrorist attacks — onto the
bridge behind me (or in front of me, or at any time before or after
I have crossed the bridge, but let's face it, while I'm on the bridge
is much worse), having failed to follow even the most basic and
fundamental security feature of the race.

I heard a squelchy reply through the walkie-talkie. I heard the
runner — a young guy, in his late twenties — pleading his case.
But that was all. That old tough-love truism of sobriety, "Better
him than me," was a boon to my spirits. I had done the right things;
he had not. At the 4.85-kilometre mark, I crossed onto the eighty-
seven-year-old super-structure of the original Ambassador Bridge.

All those kilometres logged at Malden Park, Blue Heron Park,
and in the Limberlost paid off. Running up the Ambassador Bridge
was, for me, the easiest part of the half-marathon. The air was clear
and bracing, truckers (their traffic restricted to the U.S.-bound lane
and their speed reduced to a crawl) blasted their horns in apprecia-
tion. I passed a giant named Angus who was running in a kilt. As
we descended into the Customs plaza on the Windsor side at the
6.85-kilometre mark, I was ahead of pace and feeling warmed up
and loose. Friday's run-ins with CBSA personnel were completely
forgotten, their incipient evil and officiousness completely undone
by the CBSA agents in the Windsor Customs plaza standing outside of their booths and grooving to the tunes spun by a race announcer who was standing atop an angular concrete slab used to
separate inbound traffic and speaking into a microphone.

The tubular speaker he held tucked under his arm projected his
voice — a steady stream of names of recognized runners, on-the-fly
running gear analysis, wry quips, self-deprecating jokes, and avid
encouragement — across the gentle downward slope of the plaza.
As one song faded out, his roller rink/strip club DJ's voice filled the

air: "All right, all you runners out there, we hope you're all having a good time because here comes some good-time music!"

With that, resplendent atop his plinth in a track suit that was simply too robin's-egg blue and too tight to be anything but a fashion accessory, this race-day wag performed a Robert Pollard-esque leg kick and microphone twirl before sinking into a slow, one-footed spin as the organ, bass, and brass fanfare for *The Brady Kids* hit single "Good Time Music" (go ahead, YouTube it before you read any further) filled the air.

I'm not sure what this cat's radio credentials were like, but he could hit the post like nobody's business. It was like he'd been up all night with a group of CBSAs, practising for this moment, so in tune was everyone's groove. As I ran through this set piece, heading into the sharp right-hand turn out of the Customs plaza onto north-bound Huron Church Line, my earworm for the next 14 kilometres chewed its way into my endorphin-softened brain. Friends, I didn't hate it. In fact, if I was the type of runner who ran with music, it would be on repeat.

Students from the University of Windsor residence halls at the corner of Wyandotte Street and Huron Church Line had a water station set up along the western edge of the campus. Running free and easy, with Greg and Marcia Brady leading the funky mantra of positivity to which I kept pace, I decided to throw moderation to the wind and get my fill of hydration. I tucked my tube of Body Glide into the pocket of my shorts so I could double-fist it through the gauntlet of water-bearing undergrads.

Three or four waxed cups of water later, I reached into my pocket to retrieve the Body Glide — it had become a talisman, a source of comfort; knowing that if even the slightest sting of chafing crept up anywhere on my body, I had the remedy in my hand — only to discover it was gone. I shot a quick glance back over my shoulder to see if it was in sight. But in the sea of crushed waxed cups and feet, it was gone. I've been known to stop a run mid-stride at chafe's first faint rash. *The Brady Kids*, though ... right there in my ear, grooving on the carpeted plinths of my memory of that particular episode, urged me, through song, to keep my emotions in check and keep negativity at bay. So, instead of wallowing in the horrors of what was only a potential future of friction-burned and sweat-irritated skin, I thought about what a boon my lost tube of Body Glide could be for another runner, someone somewhere in the pack behind me, just having crossed the bridge and feeling, somewhere on their body, the first blush of what could shortly become a flesh-melting inferno, only to find the plastic tube pin-wheeling in the street before them ...

I'd been looking forward to the right-hand turn onto Riverside Drive all morning. A few hundred metres east, three houses past the "5-mile" marker painted on the road, was where my friend Jeffery was going to be doling out citrus. I could hear the band playing before I made the turn. I could see a makeshift wooden stage set up on the front lawn, a bunch of young musicians chugging their way through a shambolic, though spirited, rendition of a Green Day song. The lawn had taken on something of a festival atmosphere, with spectators, family, and friends milling about, enjoying the fall sunshine and the spectacle of thousands of runners coursing by. Two tables at curbside were running with juice as Jeffery, his wife and children, and a crew of Jeffery's old fraternity brothers reduced two hundred pounds of oranges into individualized energy smiles for runners. They'd been doing it for several years running, for nothing more than the feeling they got from helping those who were putting themselves through such a grueling trial. I got my wedge of orange and threw the rind into the overflowing gutter after wearing it over my teeth and making eye contact with another runner.

Also along Riverside Drive, another feature of the post–Boston Bombing road race scene: a radiological weapons detector. Race literature had explained that these safety precautions would be found at several places along the course, but they cunningly had not specified where. Although it looked like something you would see rotating atop a naval destroyer, the detector, painted bright yellow, was mounted in the grass curbside. Every runner had to run past the detector. No exceptions. Police officers were stationed at the approach to the contraption, ushering those running under the impression that they were the exceptions, off the grass and guiding them by the arm back onto the road where they had to pass in front of the giant, radiologically sensitive beam.

There was no indication of what would happen if a runner was found to be packing a dirty bomb, or was just highly radioactive due to medical treatments (this contingency had been covered in the race literature), though I assumed somewhere nearby, in a conspicuously unmarked van, wise-cracking radiological weapons–detecting techs were downing coffees and watching monitors and getting ready to hit the panic button and close down the street. I could picture covert operatives dropping from trees, stepping out from topiary, abandoning false picnics at the feet of various public sculptures and rappelling down the side of apartment buildings at the first sign of a radioactive spike.

I hit the Canada Customs plaza (admittedly scanning the uniformed tunnel staff for my hypertense and moustachioed friend from the tote bag incident and fortunately not finding him) and made the sharp left down into the maw of the tunnel. It was time to cross back stateside.

I'm not one for heights, but when you're running over the Ambassador Bridge, you're not balanced on the rounded surface of a suspension cable. You're on a flat, two-lane concrete road that arcs gently over the river, in the wind and the sun. Worst case scenario, you can always go over the side and, if everything's tucked and cupped just so, hit the water and survive. The Windsor-Detroit

Tunnel, on the other hand, offers no such amenities. If shit goes south down there, you're not just under water, you're under the primordial muck of the riverbed. The air is being pumped down to you. Car exhaust is being pumped out. Things live in the maintenance ducts that have never seen the light of day. You enter into a gaping maw of artificial light and commercial billboards; you exit through a cloaca 2 kilometres distant in a militarized foreign land. You are bound on all sides by concrete and steel under enormous pressure; the vaulted ribs of the leviathan tubes they originally sank into the trench excavated into the bottom of the river have swallowed a rectilinear serpent of equal length, its innards tiled with yellow scales and bioluminescent esca. There is no inspirational vista. There is no horizon to speak of. There is only the nadir: the literal and figurative low point of the race.

As we entered the mouth of the tunnel, it was as if a light mist was falling, but it was just the airborne sweat of thousands, filling the subterranean space and trickling down the tiled walls, slicking everything it touched. The midway point of the Windsor-Detroit Tunnel is well known for its demarcation of the international border between Canada and the U.S.: flags of the respective nations painted on billboards affixed to the tunnel walls on either side of a black line and small benchmarking plaque mark the division between the two countries. Spotting the flags and trying to determine exactly when your body passed between the two countries while sitting in a vehicle travelling 60 kilometres per hour has long been a fun and fascinating way for children crossing the border to pass a few fleeting moments. *"Keep your eyes out for the flags, kids! Aaaaaanddddd ... now we're in another country! Fun, eh?"*

This game I just described, though, is for children, not for the peritoneal blockage of sweat-slicked runners stopping to take photos of themselves and each other standing before the flag billboards and the border's black ribbon of paint. Any runner who didn't want to come to a dead stop had to wedge themselves sideways, arms over their heads to increase their slenderness and balance in order to make it through the *en masse* photo op.

There was no deep house or old-school funk blasting from the speakers in the U.S. Customs plaza. There were no celebratory tunes or vibes of any kind, just the haggard breathing of hundreds of runners emerging from the humid uphill miasma of the last winding leg of the tunnel into the cool air and sunlight at the foot of the Renaissance Center, and the unflinching scowls of Homeland Security agents, arms akimbo or hands on pistol butts or wrapped around assault weapons. This is at kilometre 14 of the half. This was where the divergence happened: the full-marathoners turning right and heading east on Jefferson Avenue, bound for their lap of Belle Isle, the halfers turning left for the descent onto the Lodge Freeway.

Some people will stop for nothing during a race. Not for family, not for dear friends, not for a row of downy goslings crossing the course. It's nice to be focused on a Personal Best time, but it's also nice to be focused on people and how much you owe to running. For example, along with my sobriety, I owe my life and my well-being to running. I owe my family my continued involvement in both those things. Running is an investment in a multitude of futures aside from my own — from Jennifer and I growing old together, to living long enough to see the family grow as our children start families of their own, those children knowing their grandfather … these are simple, natural things. Things I always wanted but was compelled to forfeit and destroy through alcoholism and overeating. Which is why, when I spotted Jennifer and the kids leaning over the railing watching for me, I stopped.

"We found a hobo nest!" the kids informed me as I reached up to hug them. Jennifer and Nathanael told me the story of how Jonah and Thomasin, playing hide-and-seek in Hart Plaza, had discovered this "hobo nest" — a collection of coats, blankets, and cardboard in amongst the riverfront park's concrete outbuildings. In our brief encounter at the railing, they were excited to tell me about what they had learned about their discovery, why it was there, why people had no homes and lived on the streets, as if I, their sheltered father, never would have guessed that such tragic and degrading circumstances were possible. It was at once funny and sad. It was moments like this — revelations like this, of simple things I would never have noticed before — that running provided in its own humbling high realism. When I am feeling bad about my running, I just need to remember how easily I could have been living on the streets, separated from my family, gathering discarded clothes, and losing weight through malnourishment and disease, had my trajectory not changed. I often lose sight of that.

But what running giveth, the racing thoughts of the runner can take away. After running down a traffic-less Lodge Freeway, like survivors fleeing the same apocalypse that left us in our brightest, tightest clothes, the course climbed an off-ramp from freeway grade to West Lafayette Boulevard, arriving before the classic blue edifice of the venerable John K. King Books at the 15-kilometre mark before turning right and heading west, back toward the Ambassador Bridge.

This was, for me, the longest and most desolate stretch of the race — if for no other reason other than I was entering that phase of any long run where that restless boredom begins to set in. Chafe was beginning to raise its first raw plateaus, a patch I could feel extending from mid-thigh high up into my groin. The heady heights of "Good Time Music" had been replaced by a sharply focused point of pain and its associated mantra of "This fucking sucks."

From somewhere up ahead, I could hear the palsied, discordant strivings of a live band of dubious quality, chugging through another '90s radio rock cover — something that was only going to further sour my mood. As I drew nearer — somewhere between the 15- and 16-kilometre markers — they launched into a rollicking version of Cheap Trick's "Surrender," and I tell you, it brought tears to my eyes it was so gorgeous and loose and spirited. And it provided the answer to my woes, short-lived as they were: *I needed to give myself to the run.*

At this point, more than two thirds of the way through, what was the point of letting some non-fatal, physical discomfort infect my thinking and contribute to my second guessing my abilities, indeed my entire outlook toward what a few kilometres back had felt already like a triumph, a lifetime achievement? This was my willpower, the disease of alcoholism, the part that wants me dead, rearing up in a moment of vulnerability. What I needed to do was surrender. Gone were the bell-bottomed Bradys and their sunshine days, gone were the creeping thoughts of failure, inadequacy, and defeat; they were replaced, instead, by these flannel-flying anthem crushers and their message of not giving in, but not forcing it, either: just surrender. My inner thigh would heal. I just needed to stop over-thinking, stop fighting everyone and everything, especially myself. I was the hometown hero; I was the competition; I was the good guy — but most of all, I was the hateful enemy. Surrendering — admitting I was afraid, admitting I was in some pain, and letting it all go — that's where the strength was. If all of this seems ludicrously circular and delusional, then you've probably never been in the late stages of a long-distance run.

Through Mexicantown and Corktown we ran. Once-blighted tracts of burnt-out hovels and well-trafficked crack dens, these neighbourhoods were once again thriving. Families were out banging pot and pans and shouting encouragement from neat little front porches decked out just for the occasion. Attrition amongst the athletes was really starting to set in, though: I saw people crying on curbs, hobbling off the road to lean against trees holding their calves and quads. I wished them all well. I hoped they got it all out of their systems and just surrendered to whatever was thwarting them, and made their way to the finish line under whatever power and in whatever condition they could get there in.

In Corktown, there was a four-block stretch north on 8th Street, then a little one-block jog to the east. When you exit onto Michigan Avenue, you're looking down a straight shot into the heart of downtown Detroit, about 2 kilometres from the finish line. I was going to finish. I picked up the pace. It was a right onto southbound Griswold for one block before a final sharp right onto Fort and suddenly everyone was charging, we were all charging, toward the finish line archway that spanned the road and the rubber mats on the pavement that would digitally terminate the chip in our race bib, officially ending our race. I passed the giant in the kilt again. I passed a lot of people in the final 100 metres.

I crossed the finish line at 2:38:12. The crowd was deafening. Everything was in first-person, hand-held mode. A volunteer put a medal around my neck; another wrapped me in a foil blanket. Everywhere finishers wandered in a depleted stupor. We were eventually herded into cordoned rows of tables piled with chocolate milk, water, juice, power bars, cookies, and bagels. I scanned the throng for Jen and the kids as I wandered down Fort Street, chugging a chocolate milk and eating power bars, resplendent in my foil cape, part of the exodus from the finish area. I spotted them weaving through the crowd along the sidewalk on the south side of Fort Street as I approached a gap in the barrier. I collapsed into their arms. I thought about my mom. I thought about the promise I had failed to make to her in her lifetime. And I surrendered.

CHAPTER EIGHTEEN

THE REBELLION-SHAPED HOLE

IT WAS THE night of the final group run of the Fall Learn to Run Clinic at the Running Factory. The clinics had become a Monday night fixture on the family calendar. If I was working in the bookstore until six o'clock, I would close shop as quickly as possible (sometimes already having changed into my running clothes in the frightful employee washroom) and race down Wyandotte Street to the Running Factory, making it there just in time for the group run. It was my regular Monday night run: short and sweet, and steeped in the relaxed, fun atmosphere of the group-running environment. It was something I willingly participated in, yet, still, despite having been involved as a group leader for nine sessions over a two-and-a-half-year period and despite owing some of my fondest memories of my early running career to the Running Factory, its staff, the other volunteer group leaders, I continued to be bewitched, vexed, troubled by my own conflicted relationship with group running.

The two-poet running group I'd formed with Kira was ultimately an exercise in self-parody and collaborative fiction. It existed more as social media posts and text messages than it did anywhere in the physical world. Where running in and of itself had been a great bulwark against self-consciousness, running with other people still found me rushing headlong into everything I was self-conscious about.

It had very little to do with other runners. The judgment, the fear resided wholly within me. It was *my* problem. It's not that I want running to be exclusive, or that I believed it must always be a solitary pursuit, but sometimes in my attempts to fit in and be a part of a larger community (and this is true for any group or situation, not just runners and running), my shortcomings and insecurities (not just as a runner, but as a person) rear up, and I feel exposed and lash out. Not at others, but at myself. My head would be filled with interior monologues in which I rehashed my own lacks, my failings. I would indulge in self-flagellation aimed to beat me back down, to ensure I stayed in my station, to keep me separate and apart.

So, truly, being in any kind of running community leadership role is at times surprising, even to me. But I continue to be involved in the running clinics for the same reason I got involved in the first place: I know I have to give back. I know that I *owe*. And not just the Running Factory for being supportive and helpful. There is a more spiritual debt that needs to be paid. *I owe running.* I was willing to put my antipathy toward group running aside to repay that debt. And it was my hope that continued exposure to the group running scene through continued involvement with the clinics would eventually bring me into greater harmony with myself and with others.

But still, I chafed against it. The group run experiences that had bolstered my confidence and spurred me on were sometimes outweighed in my memory by a couple of LTR-night blows to my confidence. Most of these exposed how the strangely competitive dynamics of group running and my self-consciousness make for bad running partners. The night in question, an unseasonably warm night in late November 2015, five weeks after the Detroit Half, was not going to do anything to repair that relationship.

I'd spent most of my LTR tenure as a leader for Group 4, but for this particular session, there were no takers for Group 4, so the Group 4 leaders were running with Group 3. From the beginning of the session, it was clear this Group 3 was made up of a bunch of people who were more than capable of running in Group 4 but were afraid or unwilling to move up to the next level. The pace for Group 3 always seemed a bit too fast for those used to the longer, slower distances of Group 4. And this particular Group 3 was hooked on running *way too fast*. As group leaders, we tried to convince them that they could safely move up a level. Sure, moving up would mean they were running *longer*, but they would be able to adjust their pace accordingly, to something more appropriate for the distance. But there were no takers, and as the LTR Clinic is based on a "run at your own pace" principle, this over-throttled Group 3 was allowed to proceed apace.

From the Running Factory, Group 3 charged north on Prado Place, turning west onto the sidewalk at Riverside Drive, maintaining a 6:30-per-kilometre pace for the first five hundred metres. I can maintain that pace, but it's only really possible toward the end of a much longer run, when I am warmed up and well lubricated. I fell behind almost immediately. Looking at my watch about one kilometre into the run, I saw that I was barely staying out of the eight-minute-per-kilometre range. Checking the watch was a reflexive formality. It didn't tell me anything I didn't already know: I was obviously labouring to maintain a pace that on any previous run I would have considered relaxed. I felt winded, strangely distended, and mechanically unsound. I hadn't even broken a sweat, and I was already running through a mental checklist of all the possible indicators of a bad run.

Frustrated and perplexed, I watched the rest of Group 3 cross at a light some two blocks ahead of me. The route is a simple out-and-back, at the fifteen-minute mark on the run "out," everyone turns around and heads back to the Running Factory. I had a 400-metre lead on the "back" portion of the run for about ten seconds. Within about five minutes, the gap had been closed entirely and efficiently, and Group 3 went trotting past one of their own — a "leader" and LTR veteran only five weeks removed from a Personal-Best half-marathon in Detroit — sloppy in stride and huffing like a newcomer who had decided he was going to show up for the last night of the clinic and run with the big boys and girls. Brad, a long-time LTR group leader, slowed down and ran backwards for a few metres to make sure I was okay. I don't remember my answer, but it satisfied him, and he pivoted back to the fore. I was alone once again.

When I arrived back at the Running Factory, most of Group 3 was exiting the store and heading to the pub across the street, site of the traditional, end-of-session party. I spent an embarrassed few minutes stretching against the store's exterior wall. I was actually trying to think of excuses — witty rejoinders and sage deflections — because I figured that when I turned around there was going to be a lineup of LTR participants waiting to rub my nose in the fact that they were better runners than me; champing at the bit to let me know that I had been exposed. I felt exactly that — exposed. I felt like a fraud brought into the harsh light of truth. Not by the dogged work of some investigating party but by my own laziness and corpulence. Because, truly, I felt like I once again weighed 368 pounds.

That's where I was at, mentally; I was feeling that I should just go finish off the meal I balked at, almost three years ago to the day, when I was leaving the cardiologist's office. Like a fool. A fucking fool who, in his midlife crisis blindness, thought he could get sober from food, too.

It's no secret that runners are ridiculously stubborn people. There are no memberships, no gyms. The only required equipment is shoes. You lace them up, you hit the streets … and endure the one-foot-in-front-of-the-other monotony that will at once change your life for the better, and leave you exhausted, sore, and, during peak training, irritable and stressed out. It takes a lot of stubbornness to put yourself through that, repeatedly, and somehow find confidence, tranquility, and solace in what can be so painful, unpredictable and humbling. It's difficult to understand, really — what would make a person do this to themselves? It is at once monstrous, and enviable. Outside of stubbornness, most people are wont to call this particular mania willpower and hold it up as a great virtue.

As an alcoholic, I know this: it is my willpower that keeps me sick. As a runner, I found a meditative exercise that calms my mind, strengthens my body, and elevates my mood — a haven from my diseased will that paradoxically, at almost every turn, seems fuelled by willpower. Willpower is going to get me, coming and going. It's this kind of monstrous dilemma that keeps a runner of my type running, afraid to stop and lose their lone source of genuine peace and stability when they sense that maybe it's time to take their foot off the gas, to drop the mileage, to stop altogether and seek help; when the body starts to wear down because of the strain, the humbling pain of the sport. Stopping means recovery and rehabilitation. The will wants you to keep going. It wants to pound you into the ground like a stake. And when it does, your body will stop you in your tracks, despite the will urging you on and cursing your physical ineptitude. At which point, the ego, ever helpful, will top the pounded stake of your failure with a sign that reads HERE LIES

A QUITTER. Runners are ridiculously stubborn people because running requires it — a commitment that is as capable of elevation as it is of immolation.

This was the mood I was in while I was walking back to the van, unsure where I was heading but definitely not going to celebrate another successful LTR with a room full of steadily improving and increasingly inebriated runners. It was at that moment I detected underneath all the self-hatred, anger, embarrassment, and abysmal esprit de corps the cause of that night's poor performance:

I was injured. Again.

And fuck it if I hadn't been injured for weeks. And just like always (and just like just about every other runner I know), I'd been pretending the dull throb in my left hip that radiated from my glutes across my ball-and-socket, taking a little jog down into my groin before travelling down the outside of my thigh via the IT band to my knee wasn't there. I'd remained oblivious of the fact that something must be throwing off my mechanics and putting a big hitch in my stride and making it difficult for me to climb the stairs and get up off the couch. All these symptoms were the result of a weak core, a weak core I'd learned about during my first stint through physiotherapy a year before.

You'd think I would have been at least a little bit relieved, knowing that there was an identifiable cause for my poor running performance. But my despondency only deepened because if I was going to admit, finally, that I was hurt, I was going to have to admit something else: I'd gained weight. That I had been able to run the Free Press Half at 265 pounds was neither heroic nor something to be proud of when I could have run it at 225, or less. If you have a weak core, the way to work on it is not by packing on forty pounds. That's just going to increase the wear and tear and that's how you're going to end up standing next to your van after a humbling group run, staring off into space.

Running had very insidiously become the primary excuse for overindulgence. In the wake of the Detroit Half, it became too easy to let myself off the hook; it became too easy to enjoy extra helpings of supper; to eat while watching TV at night; to grab a date-filled maamoul at the Lebanese bakery on my walk to and from the book-store … It also became too easy to skip runs: *This is my off-season*, I kept telling myself. Give the body a chance to recuperate and recover from the tough summer training schedule. My metabolism had come to rely on running to such a great extent that when my mileage fell off so steeply, even small indulgences on the walk home from work a couple of times a week or an extra helping of chicken curry at supper resulted in big weight gain.

And I kept eating, and the few runs I was going on seemed that much harder: not just because my cardio had fallen off, but because I was getting heavier. It's harder to move 270 pounds than it is 265. My running clothes weren't fitting right. They were chafing against me, helping to fill my thoughts while running with self-loathing. This, too, became an impediment to running, and as my mileage fell off, motivation became harder to come by. The very thought of running became, once again — as it had been for most of my adult life — daunting. No one wants to go out a few weeks removed from a running experience that qualifies as one of the best experiences of their life only to realize they are not fit enough to run. In a fit of pique, I began to suspect that I had never really liked running to begin with. In the weeks following the Detroit Half, bad runs became the norm. My pace fell precipitously. Throw in a single shitty night at the LTR Clinic and I was finally ready — humbled enough — to admit that since late October I had been running on an injured hip and trying desperately to deny the existence of my injuries by not running and not aggravating it.

Brad came walking down the leaf-blown street and found me standing next to the van. "Are you coming to the party?"

"I don't know. I'm not much in the mood for people, or a good time."

"But there's food!" he beamed.

"I'm hurt," I said, staring off into the dark.

"Lots of people are hurt right now — it's the end of marathon season," he said. "That's why we eat all the food."

I appreciated Brad's effort to include me and followed him into the pub. The last to arrive, we were greeted with ribbing and cheers, but my enjoyment of the party, even with its rounds of appetizers and no-charge club soda, was curtailed by my smouldering despondence.

I felt I was simultaneously burning out and fading away from running.

○ ○ ○

"There will come a time," more experienced runners told me, "when you just won't want to run."

I, in turn, told them that that wouldn't happen to me. That I loved running too much. That it had saved my life, and the way I was going to repay the unpayable debt I owed was to run more, and run hard, and run with a joyful abandon.

They would chuckle, purse their lips in wry understanding, these other, more experienced runners, and they would gently reiterate their claim: there comes a time in nearly every runner's life when, not due to injury or illness or age or decrepitude, they simply cannot find it in themselves to run. What used to bring them peace and stabilize their mood will seem like a chore, an inconvenience, a mania best left on the shelf by the door with the road-weary shoes. It happens, they would say, even to them, with their racks of medals and sheaves of race bibs; their cubby-holes containing every shoe they had ever worn, each pair replete with a backstory of triumphs and defeats and a tag looped through an eyelet indicating the total distance worn.

But I am different, I maintained. My motivations for running are singular, my story the stuff of magazine features. I am, after all, writing a book about this singular and storied running career; how I identified and filled this running-shaped hole.

And despite my protests — my disbelief — it happened.

Whether it was a result of the cumulative effects of my fear of reinjuring myself or my inability to cope with running's stark loneliness — the sudden realization that I had chosen the athletic analogue to writing, in all of its monastic insularity, as my meditation, my escape, my antidote to a gastronomic suicide — my lack of interest in running kept plumbing new nadirs.

Those runners who had gently warned me to take my foot off the gas, to throttle my zeal for running a bit for the sake of my body and my peace of mind no longer seemed like buzzkills but soothsayers. They told me that when this nearly inevitable period of decline in enthusiasm for running came around, I should just take it as a sign that my body needed a break; that the universe was telling me to take a knee; that I should take heed and rest easy in the knowledge that eventually my interest in running — *my need to run* — would come back around. I would be out logging kilometres again with a renewed vigour and lightness in my step. In the meantime, I should just accept it and not be too hard on myself.

This was all solid advice. The kind of advice I intuitively knew I should take to heart because it rang true, because it coincided with what I already knew about dealing with rebellion.

Because rebellion is what this was.

I had also been told by another group of much wiser, more experienced people that the sober alcoholic, almost without exception, will at some point in their sobriety be seized by a soul sickness — *a rebellion* — so strong that even though prayer has been a cornerstone of their daily sobriety, they will simply refuse to pray. The natural tendency is to lash yourself for your obstinacy, but the alcoholic is told to not be too hard on themselves, to cut themselves some slack, and to simply resume prayer when they are able, knowing what is good for them. It would seem that acceptance of the rebellious period is a natural part of spiritual growth. But as a runner not-running, I have learned the hard way that acceptance has it limits and can be perverted, like every other natural instinct, emotion, and inclination, into the wrong kind of growth.

◦ ◦ ◦

Eventually, I was not running, and that had me oscillating between wide-eyed instability and near-somnolent disassociation. Old anxieties and fears began to recolonize my thoughts; old preoccupations from the years of overeating, obesity, and poor mental and physical health became daily visitors. I became convinced that I was going to have a heart attack, a stroke, an aneurysm, an embolism. A mysterious spiral fracture appearing after stumbling off a curb would reveal bone cancer; I was going to get hit by a car, crushed under the falling limb of a tree during tornado season. It was irrational, it was regressive, it was paralyzing … and it was stopping me from getting back in my shoes and hitting the pavement. I knew this.

This was not something I realized in retrospect. I knew this as it was happening. As my mood fell, my energy levels fell, and just like I can't write when I'm not happy, I cannot run when I am similarly disturbed.

I knew that it went deeper than the frailties of the flesh. It was tied inextricably to the unshakable suspicion that I was a fraud as a runner. And if I was a fraud as a runner, what the hell was I doing writing a book about running? The answer came all too easily: I was also a fraud as a writer. Here I was, deep into a creative non-fiction memoir about how running filled up a spiritual hole that had existed inside of me long before I realized it was there; how filling that running-shaped hole changed my life for the better and made me more confident and capable and fulfilled — and I was afraid to run, which was doing a number on how confident, capable, and fulfilled I felt. The vicious cycle of being unable to run off the stress that not running created, getting further and further away from the solution, moved me further and further from my writing. Every time I sat down to write, I would have to think about my running: When was the last time I'd run? When was the last time I'd run three times in one week? When was the last time I'd run more than 5 kilometres? And more often than not, what I was confronted with was the fact that it had been too long on all counts.

To all of this — this lack of serenity, this failure of self-confidence, this return of crushing self-consciousness — running was the answer. Everything else would fall into place if I could just bring myself to run, even just 5 kilometres every other day, whether to start, or in perpetuity. But I could not bring myself to it with any kind of surrender or grace. I could drag myself to it, once or twice a week (a feat the runners who warned me about exactly this kind of running malaise would bill as a triumph). After each of these runs, I would feel every positive thing running had ever done for me. I felt lean, lithe, and aerodynamic; accomplished and confident. I was spiritually buoyed and mentally sharp. And I would try to bring myself — *try to surrender* — to not just the acceptance that I have to do this regularly to be happy, but to the action of it, because the running clearly isn't in the knowing, it's in the doing.

The feeling of not running — to be a runner seized by this rebellion, this unclear place that isn't wholly thought but isn't wholly feeling — is the worst kind of injury. Because outside of therapy with a sports psychologist who helps athletes under more pressure than I was certainly under overcome the yips, mental blockages, career-defining errors, big losses, and the stress of high-level achievement, there was little that I could do aside from running. Running was my therapy. My meditation. My solace. My joy. And I was removed from it. Only one remove, mind you, but the distance seemed too great — a run over terrain beyond my experience, and now, clearly, beyond my fitness level. This rebellion feeds on itself. I knew all it would take is one good run — a run where the air and light mixed with my stride and my mood — for me to fall back in love with running.

It doesn't need to be pointed out (and believe me, there are people who luxuriated in pointing it out) that the longer I avoided running, the heavier and more out of shape I got. Where, for more than two years, I stepped on the scale every morning and weighed myself, recording each day's weight down to the decimal place in a logbook kept in the linen cabinet in our upstairs hallway, I hadn't stepped on the scale in months out of embarrassment and fear. In fact, the day I stopped weighing myself every day (I don't know exactly when it was but it was sometime in 2015, when I was certain that I would never face a crisis in my running life, and that I would never turn to food for comfort or out of boredom or self-consciousness again; that my weight would be under control forever) can safely be chalked up as a colossal fuck-up; the beginning of a tremendous backslide.

How is that supposed to inspire confidence — for me, or for anyone else? How is feeling weaker, more bloated, less confident, and more vulnerable supposed to make me love running? Here's something I've learned running, but only realized twenty seconds ago: running is good for depression. But depression is not good for running. It's diabolically circuitous and paralyzing.

All through the writing of this chapter, I was seized with the knowledge that the writing was not going well because I felt like I was forcing it. Forcing comparisons like this one, in which I compare forcing myself to write and forcing myself to run. Even though forcing yourself to write isn't fun, it is better than being stubborn and precious — a delicate flower who can only write under very specific and favourable conditions: not total silence, but not a wild rumpus; not the peace of early in the morning, but not the restlessness of the evening either. Has everyone been nice to me? Am I worried about someone or something? All of these injustices to my person — whether real or merely perceived — have played roles in why I haven't written when the opportunity to write is right there, waiting to be plucked like the fruit we are supposed to taste. So, if the last few hundred words, which strike me as doing a decent job of keeping with the thing I am struggling to write about — the pesky comparison between forcing myself to write and forcing myself to run — can be written in the self-imposed duress of forcing myself to write, what kind of good can come of forcing myself to run?

○ ○ ○

It's true that a problem shared is a problem halved, but when I asked my son Nathanael, then thirteen years old, to start running with me on a regular basis, I didn't so much halve the problem as I did double the number of people I was comfortable running with. I didn't tell him I had become irrationally and paralyzingly afraid to run by myself (despite my deep dislike of running in groups) because I didn't want him to know how much my enthusiasm for the pursuit that had changed my life so dramatically had waned; how tenuous my hold on stability could be in the face of that waning enthusiasm, that fear, that loneliness. And maybe that's what it really was: a fear of being out there on the streets, trails, and pathways alone.

When Nathanael had run with me in the past — and he had exhibited a fitful interest in running ever since I had started running — we didn't always have a successful run. But we always shared meaningful time together, even if it passed largely in silence. As he grew and surpassed me in height and became a young, strong man, I became more convinced that not only did we need to run together more because I wanted so badly to have someone who knew me and understood me at my side, but also because, as he entered those turbulent teenaged years, it became clear to both Jennifer and me that Nathanael needed to run for the all the same reasons I needed to run: to cope with the self-consciousness, the eating, the anxiety, the creeping depression.

In convincing Nathanael to run with me, I was able to distract myself from my fears; I told him running would make him feel better — about his physical appearance (those awkward growth phases of the early teenaged years), his school performance–related anxiety, his free-floating dysthymia. I wasn't lying. It would make him feel better if he decided to stick with it and make it a practice.

◦ ◦ ◦

Nathanael and I were making a regular habit of running together a few times a week in the late winter and early spring of 2016. We set a goal: to run the Running Factory Spring Thaw 5K together for the second time, but this time we would train together, and we would attack the course and aim for a sub-thirty-minute time. Sometimes, before our training runs, there would be tears: it was too cold; he was too tired; he just didn't feel like it. More than once, my gambit of telling him I was getting ready, and that if he was coming, he had ten minutes to meet me at the front door with his running shoes on or I was leaving without him, went completely untouched in favour of the too-tempting lures of gaming,

YouTube, and texting with friends, and I would leave for the run glum and alone. But just as often, he would lace up his shoes without complaint and we would head out together, always hugging in front of the house at the end, where he would sheepishly thank me for cajoling and bribing him into the run, and I would just tell him I loved him and thank him for running with me. And I really did love running with him. It made me feel less vulnerable and alone, but more importantly, it made me more patient with my son.

"This is good for us," I said during a long run in which we discussed *The Godfather* movies, the novels of John Bellairs that had frightened both of us so much, and some of the social pressures he was facing in high school, which, as of late, had been bothering him. "Not just the talking while running. And not just the physical benefits of the running. But the effects running has on things like mood and self-worth for people like you and me — people who aren't —"

"Out-there energy people?" he offered.

He understood, and I felt better knowing that he did. We were definitely not "out-there-energy people."

Jennifer was thrilled that we were running together. "It makes me happy when you get to do stuff with kids without me," she told me one day, when Nathanael and I had returned from a run and he had gone upstairs to shower. "You guys are always so happy when you get back," she laughed, knowing how hard it could be for us to get out the door.

"I'm trying to make up for when I stopped you from running," I said, harkening back to her cajoling me into running with her when she had joined the Learn to Run Clinic some seven years before.

Jennifer admitted she didn't know what to do with me at that juncture in our marriage. "You were just so frustrating at that point," she said. "I tried to leave the door open for you to join me, but I knew it was up to you — either you'd get there, or you wouldn't. I didn't want your frustration to derail my goals, but ..."

"And when I didn't?"

"I just loved you anyway."

Despite knowing me the way she did, knowing my self-consciousness about my weight and my all-consuming fears of dropping dead because of that weight, my adoring and compassionate wife had left the door open for me to run with her, and it was clear that in leaving the door open for me to join her, too much of the worst of me had gotten in, and she had stopped running and suffered as a result. Running with Nathanael was a small part of the ongoing amends I needed to make to my wife.

Try as I might to get Jonah, with his natural runner's frame and athleticism, interested in running — as a way to increase his confidence in school as a means to improve his ability to have success with his different style of learning that required him interact with the curriculum through the use of a tablet, which made him feel singled out and put him in the crosshairs for the cruelties of classmates; as a way to, maybe, make him hungry enough that he would try a new food (like an egg or a hamburger) — it wasn't his bag. He accompanied Nathanael and me on two runs, during which he was frustrated with our pace, running backwards, leaping over park benches and hydrants, and pulling pratfalls, never getting winded or breaking so much as a sweat. When we pulled up in front of the house, he joined us in our customary post-run hug and said, "Aaaah, this is nice. But I don't like running."

We were heading slowly up the steps onto the porch when he asked, "Dad, how do I get into parkour?"

Nathanael and I ran the Spring Thaw 5K. We didn't break the sub-thirty mark, but we finished with a big surge of adrenalin, pounding south down Villaire Street from Riverside Drive, rounding the corner hard at Wyandotte, and charging through the chute to the finish in 33:31.

I figured our joint success in the Spring Thaw was going to be the thing that melted the barrier between Nathanael and running. But even with the promise of a GPS running watch of his own dangling before him, Nathanael's interest in running waned just as precipitously as my own. Maybe I was relying too much on investing in someone else's burgeoning running career to distract myself from my own woes and fears? Maybe I corrected him too much on breathing and form and pace and made him feel inferior and perpetually out of step? Or maybe it was my extemporaneously delivered lectures on photography, or my commenting opprobriously on the state of CanLit, or my encouraging him to focus his art on his own raw, idiosyncratic style rather than on emulation and portraits of celebrities copied from magazine photos? Regardless, it was a short-lived experiment, and it was not his fault. He needs running, just as much as I do, and for many, if not all of the same reasons. But he's going to have to arrive at that knowledge on his own. Too much pressure creates rebellion, not accord.

I know because I've been there. I know because *I can still be there*. I had fallen prey to that most subtle form of rebellion: complacency. I needed to get back to basics. I needed get back to the place where my obsession with food and my very real fear of dying of obesity collided to compel me to walk twice around Willistead Park. I needed to remind myself of where I was and get honest about how easily I could go back — all the way back and beyond.

Fitful flirtations with regular run schedules and training for and, once, registering for a half-marathon that I hardly trained for and certainly didn't show up to run, were punctuated with months of inactivity. I would stand behind the bookselling counter at Quixotext and promise myself I would go for a run after work — even just a quick 2 or 3 kilometres — and nothing would happen. Everything seemed to be in a stasis.

And then one day, Thomasin's pancreas stopped working. There was a blur of nightmarish days on the pediatric ward, sleeping sitting up in chairs and on the hospital bed next to our scared little girl who, at ten, faced with the unfathomable lifetime ahead of her, each day punctuated by needles and bloodied fingertips, was coming to grips with her diagnosis of Type 1 diabetes.

Jennifer and I spent many intense hours with the pediatric nurses, whose job it was to educate us over the course of a few days on diabetes care. Thomasin was not allowed to leave the hospital until the nurses were confident we understood the very serious nature of the disease and were able to care for our daughter.

During one of these sessions, one of the nurses nodded down at my well-worn New Balances and said, "You a runner, Dad?" Bleary eyed and overwhelmed, I said that I was, but that I hadn't been running very much in the past several months.

"Well, you had better just keep on running," she said, "because this little girl needs her daddy, and you are going to need to be a good example of long-term health for the entire family."

And true to the pattern that had plagued me since the day I denied my mother the deathbed promise in a room in that very same hospital, I didn't do it. But this time, I didn't make an excuse. I just let the fear wash over me — and stay over me — like a kind of security.

CHAPTER NINETEEN

WE WILL FALL

August 23, 2017

THAT NIGHT, NATHANAEL and I went out for a run. It was a special run for a bunch of reasons. It was special because in order to get Nathanael, having recently turned fifteen, to acquiesce to the run, I had to admit to him that I wasn't exactly thrilled about heading out for a run, either; that I would rather stay home and read and listen to music and eat something (three things we both love to do!); and admit that for too long I had been using my fear of running by myself as an excuse to not run, and that tonight, with or without him, I was going for a run. It would be short; it would feature father and son in matching Running Factory running hats and New Balance 860V6s; there would be walking breaks and some actual "standing still on a street corner drinking water" breaks.

It was special because it was my second run in as many days, coming at a time when finding the motivation to run had been so painful and difficult.

It was special because earlier that day I'd finished the revisions on another draft of this book, lowering the working manuscript into a red-and-grey New Balance shoe box with THE RUNNING-SHAPED HOLE BY ROBERT EARL STEWART scrawled rakishly across the lid with a black Sharpie.

It was a special day because the next day Thomasin turned eleven, and although she was too sassy and preteen girly to join us on our run, she was happy and healthy and thriving in spite of her T1D diagnosis.

It was also special because about one hundred and twenty metres into the run, I fell. The toe of my right shoe caught a lip in the pavement on Niagara Street, a few metres off the corner of Gladstone Avenue. I went crashing to the concrete, sending a jolt of pain up my left arm when my palm struck the sidewalk in a reflexive attempt to break my fall. There was a lot of scuttling, slappy sounds. My left knee raked across the concrete's swept striations. I went into a shoulder roll, my left elbow and shoulder rasping along the ground, too.

I heard Nathanael say, "Oh shi—" before switching it, mid-utterance, to "Oh shoot!"

My first instinct upon coming to rest on the sidewalk was to assure him I was okay, even though I wasn't sure if I was. I couldn't tolerate the thought of him standing there, even for a second, wondering if this was where I would leave his world — in front of Deserault's Variety.

While I lay there on the sidewalk, telling him I was okay, that I just needed a second to make sure before I attempted to stand, I was transported back to that first Krapp Brothers adventure in the canoe at Oxbow Lake, when I was morbidly obese and afraid of dying of a massive and bloody combined cardiac-gastrointestinal event in front of my horrified and helpless children.

There comes that point in every young man's life when he sees his father for what he is: hapless, imperfect, feckless. It is every father's job, I believe, to somehow remove himself from that pedestal. I think, in this instance, with my oldest child, this was more of a reiteration of my hapless, imperfect fecklessness; a refresher course. What better way to show him than crashing in a heap onto the sidewalk on a late-night run, minutes after admitting to him (again, not for the first time) that I was emotionally weak, inherently lazy, and motivationally crippled in the face of an activity that at one time had been a legitimate lifestyle, a passion that had saved my life?

Cursory investigation of my injuries determined that I had not spiral-fractured my forearm. Though charlie-horsed in three different places, my right leg, which had borne the violent, muscle-rupturing brunt of the toe stubbing on the unseen lip in the pavement, did not seem structurally or mechanically damaged in any serious way. I wasn't even bleeding, so light was my road rash. Now it was time to show my son how an old man springs back to the task at hand.

Nathanael helped haul me to my feet. I checked my GPS watch, which I hadn't had the presence of mind to pause mid-fall, and we continued east on Niagara. Our first walk break, though, was coming early.

We walked in silence for one block, and at Lincoln Road, I decided I was unhurt and certainly not about to let my mildly abraded knee, elbow, and shoulder bring the run to a sad end, so, we picked up the pace again. A few blocks later, we turned into the main gates at Willistead Park, crossing the very patch of pavement where some thirty-eight months earlier, unbeknownst to Nathanael, I assaulted a man in the street and committed acts of mischief.

Once on the super-path, Nathanael broke our silence: "I almost swore," he chuckled.

"I know," I said. "You're lucky. You would have been grounded."

o o o

Earlier that day, when Kira saw the photos of the New Balance shoebox containing the manuscript I had posted to Facebook, she was among the first to chime in with congratulations. Of course, she asked after my running; there was no use trying to candy-coat it — I told her about how my zeal for running had cooled, how I had ignored those who cautioned me about injury and waning interest. I told her that training for the Detroit Marathon in 2014 and not being able to run it because of my legal imbroglios was not nearly as stressful and painful as training for and actually running the Detroit Half in October 2015.

I wrote, *I don't think the human body is meant to be pushed like that. Not mine at least. I don't think I'll ever train like that again. For me, 5 and 10Ks work. They don't take up all my time; they don't stress me out and make me miserable — they do for me what I need running to do for me; the stuff that got me hooked in the early days. Short, pleasant runs make me feel capable, prepared, relaxed, and confident. Training for a half and running a half every weekend for two months made me fearful, discontented, self-critical, angry, and depressed.*

All of this, I told her, was compounded by how thrown off I was by the feeling of fraudulence that came from writing a book about running, and how I was paralyzed by the enveloping fear about running itself, which was couched in pride and shame's maelstrom of self-aggrandizement and self-flagellation. I hated myself for not being able to go out this very evening and bust off a 16K. Or even a 6K, truth be told.

Kira said she had experienced the same kind of cooling. Like me, she could actually pinpoint the two running-related events that caused her interest in running to wane. *Don't be hard on yourself,* she wrote in a text message. *I think that part of running is taking a break from running. I think it gives you time for your body to heal from the training and to renew your sense of joy for it. Now when I run, I do it because I want to … I think the urge can go dormant, but it never goes away. And I wholly believe it comes back.*

She stressed, though, that she could not run in the summer's thick humidity (less punishing in Toronto than Windsor, but still oppressively muggy). The only way she could run while awaiting fall's gorgeous running climes was to run at night. How I even attempted to run in August's midafternoon heat and humidity, she said, was beyond her.

But maybe running, in general, was beyond me. Maybe a comeback wasn't in the cards. Aside from my feeling physically weak and impotent, spiritually thwarted and static from not running, I harboured fears that the manuscript I had just submitted that day was nothing more than the latest piece of evidence that I was a fraud as a runner.

○ ○ ○

Nathanael and I were midway through Willistead Park when I opened up to him about how I felt: "I think what I've written is good," I said, "but it isn't about anything I am *actually doing.* I do *not* want to be the guy who wrote a book about running but isn't a runner."

"We're running right now," Nathanael said, confused. "You always said to me that if you are out running in the streets and it's not some kind of cataclysm or emergency then you are a runner."

He was right, of course. I did say that. But where I upheld it as the truth about other people, did I believe it as the truth for me? Wouldn't the more principled and honest way to live be, if I was trying to sell someone a line about focusing on light 5Ks and finding a way to enjoy running again, to not approach it with such trepidation? Maybe I should start by putting some of those words into practice, cut myself some slack and allow myself to ease back into running without running under respiratory duress. Hence this night run, where my poor night vision led me to prostrate myself on the pavement in front of my son.

"Maybe," Nathanael said, "finishing the book is helping you like running again. Maybe you should just stop thinking about your running in terms of the book all the time and just keep running."

This kid is only fifteen years old, I thought as we headed south along the super-path, continuing onto Kildare Road down toward Shepherd Street. It was there that I realized that tonight's fall — a fall that could very easily have resulted in me breaking my wrist, totalling my knee, and wrecking my shoulder and hamstring but instead did none of these things; a fall that happened in the lingering halcyon glow of having, earlier that day, submitted the manuscript for this book; a fall preceded a few hours before by a text message conversation with an old running friend, encouraging me to run at night — served a higher purpose.

Aside from the obvious symbolism of falling — it being the result of the hubris of overtraining and ignoring the advice of other runners, and as a result getting injured and becoming disillusioned with running and coming down, hard, from those first few years of over-zealous rapture — there is also the terminal point of falling to consider: there is a bottom of the downward trajectory. Like a good alcoholic, I have to learn things the hard way. Things like: sometimes, even in sobriety, there is another bottom to be plumbed and colonized with my ego and fear, and then, in classic alcoholic form, wallowed in.

I stopped running, I gained weight, I was simultaneously ashamed and too proud to start at the bottom again. But that's where I was — that's where I was, sitting on the sidewalk, in mild physical pain and jolted into the realization that I was in the most emotional pain I had been in since before losing one hundred and forty pounds through running. And like a good alcoholic, when I am in enough pain, that's usually when I will make a decision, when I will change.

This fall, this bottom in running, was necessary. It got me to a place where I was ready to actually take action against my inactivity, my torpor. Like pounding a vessel on the ground to make its contents — flour, sand, liquid concrete, or writerly thoughts — settle, this fall helped jar things into place. It gave me perspective. It helped me figure out what I wanted to say in the conclusion to this book.

Had tapering back my running to the near cessation point been necessary to completing this book? Knowing the answer to that isn't going to change anything, but I can say this with some certainty: submitting the bulk of the manuscript went a long way toward short-circuiting that fraudulence loop. It made me feel like less of a fraud as a writer, which immediately freed me up to feel like less of a fraud as a runner.

○ ○ ○

Writing about the problems in my running life was illuminating, but the illumination didn't necessarily translate into running. Only running does that. Running isn't the problem; I am the problem. Running is the solution, and the solution is change. I've learned that lesson before, the hard way. Learning it again is, possibly, even harder because now there is expectation attached. Because the running-shaped hole has memory.

I remembered things about running I had, in a matter of months, managed to forget. Remembered the simple joys of mist rising from the Detroit River at dawn, the metropolis beyond peering intermittently through the vale; the tunnel of light projecting from my headlamp revealing a flurry of insects flitting across the sweetgrass-scented trails along the Grand Marais Drain in Remington Park on a sauna of an August night; being the first set of footprints in fresh snow, seemingly in an entire neighbourhood; realizing I've run 2 kilometres and had no recollection of what I saw or felt, outside of a powerful blankness, along the way; getting lost in the looping madness of Black Oak Heritage Park after sundown in the snow; running a Personal Best at any distance; tacking a heedless 2 kilometres onto the end of a run, just because it would hurt that much more and feel that much better in the end; the potency of confidence; the humility of accomplishment; and the gratitude at finishing any run when I was once so close to death ...

Remembering all of this made me feel like running was a possibility in my life again. And with each rediscovery, I receive reaffirmation that running is a place I go to, that filling that running-shaped hole is what helps me fall in line with God's will for me; that I did not have to be ruled by fear and pride and shame. I am shown, once again, that I am naught but a humble servant; that I can be patient with myself and fall in love with running for a second time.

At night, when I set my running clothes out on the dresser and set my alarm for that early morning run, I will say a prayer before I sleep and when I wake. I will say thanks for the reminder of how tenuous all of this is, how it is all dependent on my willingness to turn my fears and my will over to a God of my understanding. I will pray for the patience that will allow me to enjoy the simple difficulty and the sublime complexity of running. And I will say thank you for the ability to run, without which this all could have been so different.

You can't fall while running if you're not out there running. Maybe the best thing I can show someone — anyone who's watching me, anyone who reads this — is what I try to show my son every time we run together: that I have to work at this stuff. I have to struggle, not against some ideal of perfection, but against my own fears, doubts, dislikes, my very personality. I have to accept that I am just a flawed person. My running is just as susceptible to these flaws as anything else. To have any success with running, I have to risk falling.

And sometimes I fall. Sometimes we fall.

ACKNOWLEDGEMENTS

THE NAMES OF some people appearing in these pages have been changed for obvious reasons, some for reasons more obscure. Other people appear as themselves.

For encouragement, camaraderie, and kilometres: Jane McArthur, James Grant, Ben Cattaneo, Kira Kovacs, Joe LaBine, Matt Daley, Clayton Klaver, Anastasia Adams, Georges Charron, and, above all others, my son Nathanael Stewart — the short list of people I actually like running with.

Joe Bertuccio, Kyle McCamon, Brad McFayden, Vicki Drysdale-Lalonde, Ingrid Kerker-Lutsch, Andrew Aguanno, Jeff Lindsay, Gary Belanger, Kelly Steele, and everyone at the Running Factory and the Learn to Run Clinics. I do love you.

Thank you to the Ontario Arts Council for its generous support of this project.

Sean Grayson is one of my oldest friends in the world. He is also a lawyer, and when called upon, he was generous with his time, counsel, and a few strongly worded letters on my behalf. Thank you, Sean.

Ellie Hastings read every page of the earliest drafts of chapters and offered editorial advice, support, and most of all, friendship. Thank you, Ellie.

Janice Zawerbny was one of this book's early champions. Her editorial hand helped point the way, and I am grateful for her guidance and insight. Thank you, Janice.

My agent, Sam Hiyate, has done more than enthusiastically represent my work. Along with his editorial assistant, Zoé Duhaime, Sam gave me a pathway and the courage to follow it, shaping and honing this story. I am blessed to have people like Sam and Zoé in my life. Thanks to them and everyone at The Rights Factory.

My editor, Dominic Farrell, was exactly the kind of presence this book needed to bring it into the home stretch. His patience, exacting eye, and his ability to guide me toward a better book were invaluable. He asked me one day, "What is more difficult, running a half-marathon or editing a book with me?" My answer: "They are both very rewarding." Thank you, Dominic.

When we were both at different places in our lives, I told Scott Fraser about this book while sitting in a London, Ontario, hotel suite, waiting out a blizzard. I'm glad I did. His interest in this book and his commitment to seeing it published have helped me move forward in ways beyond writing and publishing. To Scott and everyone at Dundurn Press — Jenny McWha, Laura Boyle, Kristina Jagger, Heather Wood, Chris Houston, Sara D'Agostino, Elena Radic, Kathryn Lane — thank you.

My wife, Jennifer, and our children, Nathanael, Jonah, and Thomasin, experienced living with me when I could not run and then had to live with my frequent absences — even while we were on vacation — while I was doing the running that saved my life and came to form the foundation of this book. Jennifer and the kids appear throughout these pages, watering me, feeding me, and offering me support and encouragement over thousands of kilometres. And even when they weren't right by my side, I was only ever running away from them so I could turn around and run back, because I knew they would be waiting for me. With love.

ABOUT THE AUTHOR

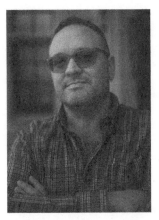

ROBERT EARL STEWART's first collection of poetry, *Something Burned Along the Southern Border*, was published in 2009 and was shortlisted for the Gerald Lampert Memorial Award for best first book of poetry in Canada. It was followed by a second collection, *Campfire Radio Rhapsody*, in 2011. His poetry has appeared in magazines, journals, and anthologies in Canada, the U.S., and the U.K., including *This*, *Magma Poetry*, *Poetry Super Highway*, *Nthposition*, *Monday Night*, *Iota*, *Moosehead Anthology*, and *The Best Canadian Poetry 2012*. He spent fifteen years as a newspaper reporter, photographer, and editor at the *Windsor Star* and the *LaSalle Post*, and has spent time as a creative writing instructor, a photography instructor, and the manager/bookseller at an indie bookstore. He lives in Windsor, Ontario, with his wife and their three children.